Soulful Pregnancy

A life-changing guide to creative & empowering pregnancy

ALICE GRIST

WOMANCRAFT PUBLISHING

Published by Womancraft Publishing, 2024
www.womancraftpublishing.com

ISBN 978-1-910559-92-5

Soulful Pregnancy is also available in ebook format: ISBN 978-1-910559-91-8

Cover design, interior design and typesetting: lucentword.com

Cover image © Niki Cotton
Illustrations © Lucy H. Pearce

Womancraft Publishing is committed to sharing powerful new women's voices, through a collaborative publishing process. We are proud to midwife this work, however the story, the experiences and the words are the authors' alone. A percentage of Womancraft Publishing profits are invested back into the environment reforesting the tropics (via TreeSisters) and forward into the community.

Praise

A profound and valuable book about the spiritual journey that is pregnancy. Alice's own account of each of her three pregnancies honours and acknowledges the individuality of each journey and encourages the reader to lean into her own experience.

Ashlyn Gibson, author of *Creative Family Home*, founder of blessstories.com

A gift to mums-to-be, supporting them to dig deep, listen to their intuition and realise the capabilities of their superpowers as a mother.

Emma Benyon, founder of Isabella and Us, editor of *Positive Wellbeing Zine for Mums*

This empowering take on one of life's most transformative journeys captures the magic and creative potential of pregnancy. Alice is the inspiring yet grounded voice I wish I'd had when I first became a mother. I'll be buying this book for all my pregnant friends.

Emma Howarth, author of *A Year of Mystical Thinking*

Through soulful, creative, and meditative practices that honour your changing body, changing life, and changing identity, Soulful Pregnancy, *will help you journey through your pregnancy feeling supported, connected, inspired and nurtured, day by day and week by week. It is magical and powerful, gritty and divine, just like you.*

Molly Remer, author of eleven books, including *Walking with Persephone, Whole and Holy, Womanrunes* and *The Goddess Devotional*

Contents

OPENING

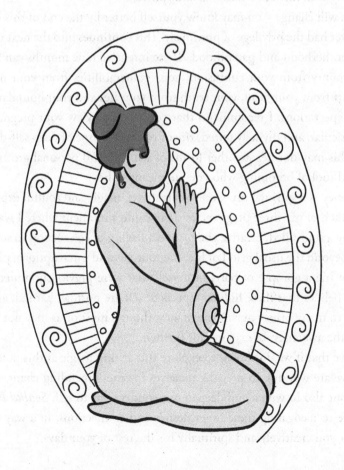

Pregnancy is a one-way trip to deep self-knowing, if we allow it. Whilst men traditionally had initiations and heroic missions, women have had periods and gestation, labour and menopause. These are some of our marks of honour and rites of passage.

People pay good money for years of ongoing therapy, self-help books, spiritual growth workshops or trips to the jungle to discover their soul through plant medicine. It is my belief that you can equally discover yourself in pregnancy, and the intention to do so makes this adventure even more powerful.

For nine months you are on a transcendental initiation to clarity. For nine months you are mostly free from addictive behaviours, stimulants and mood-altering substances. For nine months you are in your body in ways you may never have been present before. For nine months how you treat yourself seemingly matters more, for you are carrying precious cargo. For nine months others are obscenely interested in how you are, and if you are lucky, looking after your needs: physical, mental, emotional and spiritual.

Things will change. You may know yourself better by the end of this trip than you've ever had the privilege of previously. This continues into the next initiation that is motherhood and parenthood. These intensive nine months can help sort your certainty from your confusion, your vulnerabilities from your nonsense, your heart from your head, your truth from your lies and your boundaries from others' expectations. I recommend that you begin to view your pregnancy as a very particular, and divinely gifted, rite of passage, a time of deep self-discovery. Whilst this may not negate other forms of self-care and personal growth, it is a profound tool of becoming who you are meant to be.

Pregnancy is a spiritual time, one of creativity, magic and soulful exploration. Within each of my three pregnancies there came a moment where I was utterly fuelled by a soul-filled, creative energy and a feeling of connection to something 'more'. Beyond the usual grind of life, the routines and interruptions, pregnancy has given me a glimpse of parts of myself that were previously muted. I have come to believe that these hidden aspects of self are normal, natural, and likely to occur to many others during pregnancy, though most of us may not have the tools or the awareness to explore this further.

I believe that if we do choose to explore this arising magic at this potent stage of life, we are working to prepare ourselves for the impending changes of parenting, but also to widen and deepen our connections to self. *Soulful Pregnancy* is a guide to navigating these inner desires and connections, in a way that will empower you creatively and spiritually for the rest of your days.

The magic of pregnancy may not be immediate of course, there are other hills to climb first, such as sickness, anxiety, mind-boggling exhaustion, and the confirmation of that first scan. Yet, in time, with each of my three children I have found those more difficult feelings giving way to something more profound: an energy that is resilient and that demands my attention and action. The usual ebbs and flows of my monthly cycle give way to a steadier flow of vivacity (only interrupted in spates by moments of nausea and of tiredness).

This constant uplift of energy feels spiritual in nature, creative too. It is like a moment out of ordinary time, where I am infused with a desire to do. I become abundant in ideas, and the whole world feels different, more accessible somehow. It has its own unique momentum, unlike anything I have known outside of pregnancy, and it urges me into thought and action I might not usually entertain. Questions that have dogged me for months, years even, find answers overnight, and the access I have to some inner genius is closer to the surface. Beyond this I feel an urge to paint, to write and to grow things, it is like a compulsion with no end. It serves me with life skills, insight and so much fulfilment. It is the best kept secret and most profound side-effect of pregnancy.

Within all the empowerment of pregnancy there is chaos too. No matter how gracefully we tread our pregnancy path, it is likely we will be challenged. It is in these challenges that we find the fodder for our own greatness, eventually. This is something that must not be overlooked. We may wish to pass through nine months, carried by angels, as if elevated above humanity. Yet, the grit of humanity does not evade us, indeed, it may come in buckets, shovels and ways that frustrate. Let us not overlook how important this drama can be in forging us forward, and in producing power we did not know we had…

As you walk through your pregnancy, I expect your experiences will be unique and different to my own, though equally as powerful. This hot house of possibility may have been affectionately termed 'nesting' or even 'the glow' by a culture that gives little thought to the side effects of pregnancy beyond what is painful or visible. Yet it is within this space that we house the possibility for superpowers we hadn't realised we were capable of, and the resilience and determination to experiment, take risks and be, surprisingly, our most brilliant selves.

About Me

I am the mother of three, though as I write this the third is still gestating. The energy of this third child pulls me into this book, this creative and spirited exploration of what pregnancy has been and currently is for me. It's a book I would have loved to have written eleven years ago with my first child, if only I had the words. It has taken a path of further pregnancy, spiritual living and everyday magic and difficulties of life unfolding over the last decade to find the story and messages that this book holds. Writing spiritual books and teaching spiritual skills has been my passion for almost two decades. I was introduced to these subjects as a child, first through the church, when my father was an Anglican vicar, and onward to his crisis of faith that led to him become a Wiccan, and in time teaching me so much about a spiritual life that I have gone on to explore through my own lens.

Over the years I have taught many people how to work with the spiritual elements of life, using tools such as tarot, spiritual healing, intuition and to some degree psychic ability. For centuries such 'arts' have been held as skills that only specially gifted people might hold. It is my belief that we are all capable of accessing these tools within ourselves, and that imagination is a fertile spark point for such understandings and phenomena.

My background is in tarot: I have written books, created card decks, taught tarot and read for thousands of people. This is not a tarot book, but the cards are mentioned a few times in this book. If you are unfamiliar with tarot, you may have fear around them… It is part of my life mission to unfurl people's understandings around tarot, to see them as a friendly tool that the soul can wield lovingly and peacefully. The stereotypes about their demonic or dangerous background come from fear, and the unwillingness of our traditional structures to let everyday people wield spiritual insight and power in their hands. My books, cards and teachings can take you further on that path, you may wish to begin with my transformative guide to tarot, *Dirty & Divine*.

My promise to you is that the cards help you to create your life (not predict it) and that they help you explore your hopes and potential in beautiful ways. You may wish to explore a deck, or perhaps a gentler oracle deck, as you navigate your pregnancy. There are also other amazing spiritual tools you can pull in alongside this path, such as astrology, numerology, human design or practices such as reflexology, acupuncture or a form of healing such as reiki.

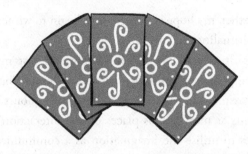

This book came to life because I wanted to share the skills of creativity and spirituality that I teach in my working life, to the people who could most benefit from them. I believe that being in a pregnant state you are ripe and ready for this heightening of self and exploring new lived experience. As you meander through pregnancy, towards inevitable great transformation, this book provides vital reflection and opportunity for growth and new understanding. This book combines all my favourite things, motherhood, spirit and creation, finding you at this trigger point of magical change, and helping to make it accessible, understood and real.

Pregnancy tends to lend itself to the experiences of sacred mystery, regardless of our previous religious or spiritual experiences or beliefs. Our connection to a soulful path is carved deep and imagination is a space wherein we can start to explore the depths of self.

For me creativity is deeply connected to our soul...but it can get switched off as we focus on chasing qualifications, material necessities and working hard at adult life. Many people I know declare too quickly that they are not creative. Favouring their logic, business skills, or formally accredited talents above anything else. Yet creativity is not to be written off so casually. It is the way you care for others, the expression you allow yourself in tone, voice and clothing, it is the way you craft calm from drama or knock up the most delicious feast from limited ingredients. Creativity is in your veins, and it is liable to come to the surface and demand exploration as you move through pregnancy and parenthood. You need not be a good artist, dancer, or writer for this to ring true. Creativity is yours to define with freedom; you can create within your life on very basic and simple levels. Allow the possibility of your own personal creativity to bubble and shimmer through you as this book offers you tasks and explorations. Take a little space for that inner creative to find their foothold.

For me, the creative imagination is the catalyst point of deep inner knowing. It is a tool of the divine, a spur to magic. Imagination is a place that, once opened, allows for evolution and great expansion. When we allow our minds to free flow, without pressure, great shifts can come.

In our time together, my hope is that you can begin to witness and experience the collision of spirituality and creativity.

At times on a spiritual path, we may feel like we are just 'making things up'. That because it happens in our minds, it is therefore imaginary and untrue. I have come to a crossroads in my understanding that honours these imaginings and made-up events as messages, as places of real interaction with the divine. Allowing ourselves to utilise the imagination as a communication point with spirit is a huge gamechanger.

As I work with spirituality, I encourage my students and clients to let these imaginings be something real, to trust them, and to light up that part of their brain that got so squashed in school. As you move forward, trust that imagination holds keys and cues to tackling life in powerful ways, and at times, to simply feel connected.

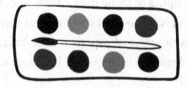

In my first pregnancy, I picked up a paintbrush for the first time since doing art at school some sixteen years previously. I created a flurry of rather poor paintings but began, over time, to learn and create with some skills in watercolour. Perhaps this was prompted by the artistic child within me – I continue to paint with her at times of much needed connection. I wrote a book in that first pregnancy and flourished in unexpected ways creatively, baking cakes and growing the most tremendous batch of tomatoes that I have yet to replicate!

My first pregnancy was joyful. It was idyllic and blissful. As far as I was concerned, I was the only woman who had ever been pregnant and therefore I skipped through each day certain of my goddess like status. The end was hard, a traumatic induced birth by forceps, that was thankfully met with a healthy child.

My second pregnancy, which was more challenging, seemed to contain the creative energy until post-birth, which then bubbled out in early maternity across the creation of a deck of cards and the writing of my book, *Dirty & Divine*. This kickstarted my career after some stagnancy and catapulted me into a whole new level and understanding of self. The stresses and strains of that pregnancy allowed for a heightening of my connection to the divine (all that is god/goddess/higher consciousness – name it what you will). Through intense and distressing events, and an empowering birth, I saw clearly that my life is not lived alone, and that I was connected to influential and loving invisible forces. If I was spiritual before that pregnancy, confirmation was given to me through the miracles and daily magic that this second child brought in her wake.

My third pregnancy, unfolding as I write this, unexpected and in many ways profoundly meaningful (finding me in difficult times), sees me revisiting my passion of writing in sudden enthusiastic bursts of energy, whilst also enveloping a new fascination with the colours on our walls (something I have studiously avoided for years – right now they would all be pink if I had my way!) ·

This book came about because of my own surprise third pregnancy at the age of forty-four. I had decided the previous year that the pregnancy window was closed for me, so this happening was a shake, rattle and roll. Whilst the child was wanted from the moment I took the test, it was not an easy thing to accept or settle into. This scenario fell at an extremely challenging period. My grandma had died a few days before the pregnancy was revealed. I had a horrible bout of illness which left me low emotionally and physically for a month or so into pregnancy. My husband was struggling with his wellbeing in a way I hadn't seen for some years. It all felt increasingly dark, lonely and frightening. Made more so by a dwindling parental support network which ten years previously had been so much more buoyant and capable.

In my anxious state I perceived doors and windows of opportunity, that had not long opened, begin to close. My own fear and anxiety nagged me. I felt compelled to tell everyone my age as if it were an apology, or in seeking out their permission. I was messy there for a while. It became a part of my creative and soulful work in the first trimester to accept my situation, to honour it, to find hope and eventually deep excitement, all the while crossing fingers and toes that nothing untoward would happen due to my grand old age.

Intriguingly, in this third pregnancy, I am a cauldron of solutions, I go to bed in confusion at what has bubbled up during the day, and I wake with the most astounding knowing and answers. Problems which I may have sat on for years are effaced by unexpected clarity. Pregnancy, it seems to me, this third time round is an opportunity to be myself all over again, to see things from a height-ened perspective, it is a sacred return to what has been forgotten, my worth and expectations of myself. Above all it is fostering trust: in my intuition, my abilities and my place in this life as a creative, spiritual, everyday mother. This I wish for you too.

How to Use this Book

My intention for this book and its activities are that they fit easily into your life and supplement and enhance your existing spiritual and creative practices – whatever they might be.

For practical purposes I have created a week-by-week guide, with all weeks of pregnancy covered. As you may not come to this book till later in your pregnancy, you may wish to revisit the early weeks at any other time, when you have a moment. The energies explored in the early days are valuable to repeat and visit whenever you wish to welcome soothing soulfulness in. Every week's theme and practices can be carried into birth and beyond into parenthood.

Each week gives you an introduction to the theme and some reflections on it, then a Meditation, a Soulful Practice, a Creative Practice, Journal Prompts and an Affirmation. I recommend that you:

- Read the week all the way through at the beginning of the week.

- Make a header in your journal with the week's title.

You may want to read through the Meditation and follow it from memory or record it on your phone and play it to guide you. If so, use a slow and calm voice, leaving gaps for meditative reflection. You may choose to use a calming music and headphones when you meditate or just do it in a quiet space. A partner or friend may enjoy reading it aloud to you. Alternatively you can access my recordings of each meditation at my website www.alicegrist.co.uk

The Soulful Practice offers spiritual tools and techniques to help you practice the week's topic in your own life.

There is very little you need to buy to do the Creative Practice activities. They are invitations to try to engage with the week's topic in a medium you are familiar with, to try new creative media when this feels exciting, to find ways to practically embed the week's learning in your life: what we do with our hands and bodies stays in our hearts.

With the Journal Prompts allow yourself at least fifteen minutes at some point in the week to consider them and write down your responses.

With the Affirmations you may wish to simply read it in your head, but the following are more powerful ways to bring it into your life:

- Adapt it to truly speak to your soul.

- Read it aloud three times.

- Write it on a Post-It note and stick it somewhere you will see it every day – your bathroom mirror or your fridge perhaps.

- Speak it aloud every morning when you are getting ready for the day.

- Write it in your journal. Decorate it with colour and doodles.

As well as a journal in which to write down your insights and reflections, I highly recommend you find a space in your home which you can dedicate as an altar space. Several weeks have suggestions specifically for this altar, and you may also wish to use it as a place to display some of the things you create during your Creative Practice activities.

You do not need to be religious to use an altar, it is simply an appointed place that you can display, reflect on and work with seasonal, sacred and special items.

An altar space might be a small table, windowsill, ledge, shelf or nook. Decide how public or private you want it to be, this will help you decide on its location. If you think it is somewhere that you would like to light a candle or incense, make sure this can be done safely in your chosen space.

For All Pregnancies

I understand that not all pregnancies are greeted with ease or levity, and that pregnancy can bring enormous physical and emotional upheaval and struggle.

With my second pregnancy, I was hauled in for more scans than I care to remember due to the baby's nuchal scan showing issues. In the end she was healthy with only a minor diagnosis that so far has not affected her life. Yet that time of being placed in grief rooms, and warned of unviability, sticks to me now. I know that place, and I dread it deeply. I don't remember much about that pregnancy. I was in a whale-like daze due to excess water and the other list of concerns that this raised. This third pregnancy arguably my healthiest, has because of my age, been prone to fearful possibilities from medical staff and intimidating tests. It has also been a journey accompanied by tricky domestic circumstances and much change and at times some instability. Pregnancy is not always the 'glow up' dictated by our culture.

Though I have some experience of the severe ups and downs of pregnancies, I appreciate that my experiences are not nearly as difficult and challenging as many others. This book cannot circumvent those harder circumstances, though I do hope it will offer solace and warmth when things are hard.

You might be experiencing any of the following:

- Facing pregnancy without a partner

- Struggles with a partner

- Pregnancy from an abusive partner or rape

- Loss of a mother or other familial support

- Extreme health repercussions: hyperemesis gravidarum, gestational diabetes, not being able to take your medication to manage chronic conditions

- IVF journey and related concerns

- Donated sperm or eggs

- Surrogacy

- Multiple pregnancies

- Struggling with addiction or an eating disorder

- Neurodivergence

- Being gender diverse

- Previous miscarriage(s)

- Previous stillbirth or sudden infant loss

- Previous abortion(s)

- Previous traumatic birth experience or a very ill baby

- Fear of birth or hospitals and/or medical practitioners

- Sadness at not being able to have the sort of birth you want

- Pregnancies in quick succession

- Financial, legal or employment instability.

Whilst I cannot speak for each one of these experiences myself, the intention of this book is to help bring you home to yourself. Not to bypass your reality or fears, but to offer a place within which to fall and, at times, to process your concerns.

Soulful Pregnancy is a deep dive into your soul. The focus within these pages is the rediscovery of the sacred, creative and powerful parts of you that exist in spite of the experiences you may have had and that you live through as pregnancy unfolds. This book will help you to access that and, growing along with your child, it will help you to be who you need to be in this moment (which is as unique as a fingerprint). The creative and soulful practices we embrace will carry us through a whole spectrum of emotion, always seeking for the possibility and magic that lies within.

Finally

This book provides a week-by-week guide to making the most of this incredible moment in time. There is no right or wrong about how your personal brand of magic may arise within you. For some it may be a whole house overhaul and socks organised in a perfect colour coded system. Others may find they take steps to grow and burgeon their careers, moving from stagnant to profound in a few short months. Many of us will find pleasure in exploring nature, taking up a new hobby, feeding a personal interest or committing to that creative outlet we have put off for years. No matter what form it takes, trust that the soulfulness and creativity will find you. The exercises in these pages will help you to hone and harness your desires, whilst also honouring and creating a lifelong exploration of truly embodied spirit and personal growth for yourself and your growing family too.

If some weeks you don't feel it, it becomes too hard, then give yourself grace. There is no one size approach here. Revisit the practices when you feel that you can.

Soulful Pregnancy is an ode to the person you are becoming and provides no pressure to conform to any standard or any cultural norm of what pregnancy 'should' be. The exercises will lead you to a trusted inner place, one in which I pray your difficulties are surmountable and you can meet your inner magic.

FIRST TRIMESTER

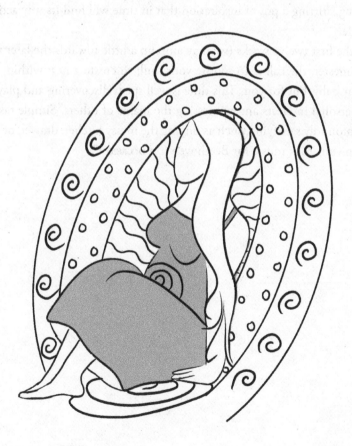

For the first few weeks of your earliest trimester, you may not even realise that a child dwells within. By the time you do find out you may hurtle swiftly into the rigours of nausea and tiredness. Even those who float easily through these early weeks may have more on their mind than a headlong passageway into soulfulness allows. As such the content we explore in these pages will begin slow and easy. Consider these early days to be an invitation, a chance to live simply and open your heart to receive the genius that you may later have the energy to pursue.

Living in a fast-paced world we often believe that creation, spirituality, and creativity must be active doing words. Yet these concepts dwell within the time we give ourselves to dream, the music we listen to, the books we read and films we watch. Each choice we make, even in our own entertainment, is an act of empowerment. So, as you move slowly through these early weeks, let your choices be a siren song to the cauldron of life that you are only beginning to gently stir.

Take this all as slowly as you can. Soulfulness can be a passive word, a place of receiving, stirring a pot of inspiration that in time will find its way actively into your life.

For the first twelve weeks (we may amp up a little towards the later weeks) of this trimester, the call is to soothe your soul: to create a nest within, not only for your baby, but for you. This time is well spent discovering and playing with your personal interests and witnessing the magic of others. Simple tasks might feel profoundly satisfying, such as tidying the messy kitchen drawer, or choosing to swap your rock music for Beethoven (on occasion!).

Weeks 1–4

Releasing the Past, Embracing the Future

It is in these first weeks when miracles happen. Beyond your vision, somewhere inside, a spark meets another and, in this instant, everything changes. In this four-week period you silently and invisibly move from singular self, into something other. This is the quiet time when your life fuses irretrievably with the life and light of another being. All of this happens unseen, away from your everyday knowing and at times, beyond all expectations.

We begin with the strange chunk of time at the start of your pregnancy that classifies your last period as week one. This is a space in which you are, for some of the time, not pregnant at all, and after that, you simply may not know it. Remarkably, you begin the first week of the forty weeks of pregnancy with the first day of your period. As such, we begin our pregnancies with a loss of the previous month's possibilities: a cleansing release. This release feels like the exact opposite of what pregnancy is: our monthly blood. It is this release that creates space, it conjures a fertile arena in which something very small may take root. But first, before that happens our bodies must shed, let go and remove the old.

The moment of pregnancy does not occur at conception, but in this story, it begins with a clearing. Similarly, when you think of a farmer's field, it may seem apparent that the life of the crop begins upon sowing of the seed. Yet there has been a time of preparation before that seed is sown that is deeply important. This usually involves a turning over of the earth, churning the old into the new, raising up the soil to make it airy and ready. Perhaps too there is the furrowing of paths for the seeds to be sown and a laying of nourishing compost. In this process the old and worn is removed, weeds and latent stock unfurled from the ground. The start begins much before the start is conceived or known.

Take this further back even. How might your pregnancy have been conceptualised

15

long before the seed took root, before the shedding of the old lining of the womb? Did it begin as a thought? As a hope? As a heartfelt plea? As a possibility you toyed with and eventually thought: YES!? Did it begin when you were an egg inside your mother's ovary, whilst your mother was still forming in your grandmother's womb?

For those whose pregnancy was not planned, was unexpected, untimely, how might we shed the expectations of what we thought life would look like to be with this moment, to accept it, to recognise that sometimes, the plan does not have to be our own for it to be accepted and embraced?

It is interesting to think on this: for the first week of every single cycle you have ever had, you are potentially in the first week of pregnancy. And yet for most of those cycles, the womb will release its lining, will shed and nothing more will be thought of it. To find yourself here, observing this beginning, one that starts with total clearing, we begin with the true spiritual power that is release.

 ## Meditation: *Release*

Start by placing one hand to your heart, and one over your womb. Take three lovely deep breaths. Imagine your energies dropping into your heart, your womb, your warm inner self. If any anxiety or stress makes itself known, imagine breathing purposefully into this space, feeling the breath begin to carry it away.

Continue breathing consciously as you spiral your attention inwards to the feelings within your body. How does your body feel right now? Are there tensions, pain or tightness? Notice each little space of discomfort and envision that the tensions and pains are little black balls. As you breathe, you purposefully release and relax these areas, the little black balls begin to roll away, carried by your breath, released to be reframed and recharged.

Now bring your attention to your mind and heart. Become aware of tight areas of anxiety, stress or worry. Feel these out and locate where they sit within or around you. Envision these areas as gatherings of little black balls. Breathe deeply, imagining the breath is being carried to the balls, which immediately start to dissipate and release under the power of your attentive and empowered breath. Breathe them out and relax a little deeper.

Drawing your attention to silence for a moment, see what bubbles up. I invite you to search within for hope: for hope is the antidote to any anxieties or fears that plague you. Imagine the hope as a bright beaming ball of light within you. Focus on how it feels within. Allow it to grow and expand, moving from some inner place to the edges and surfaces of your body, beyond that out into the air around you, until you are engulfed and surrounded by the astonishing and buoyant energy of hope. As hope takes over, you feel the release of anything toxic, anything that is not serving you. The hope pushes out the old, and opens a passageway to more of the same, hope, hope and more hope.

Let hope flush through your system, warming you and creating a higher mood, elevated understandings and allowing you to start to access the voice of hope that resides within you. Stay with this for as long as you like.

When you are ready, connect to your body, take a long deep breath. Take a few moments to breathe and stretch before returning to your day.

Repeat this meditation as often as you like.

Soulful Practice: *Release*

The beginning of pregnancy requires so many changes. Some of our most beloved crutches are taken from us and we are left feckless and de-caffeinated for some time. This too is part of the purging that is necessary. However, it does not always come easy. The early days may take some getting used to, as our morning drink is replaced, our evening drink doubtless replaced too, a penchant for sugar curbed, a desire to 'be good' encouraged. In part, the joys we have known are stripped back, and depending upon where you find your joy, this might be deeply perturbing. Yet pregnancy is release, and it is change. Our Soulful Practice this week is to honour that change with a simple ritual.

All you need is a piece of paper and a pen. Write at the top, "I welcome this change. To make space for this transition I release the following..." Then list the parts of your life you are willing or forced to say goodbye to at the present time. Focus only on what you are releasing right now, the familiar and loved parts of life that for some time you will have to reduce or release. When your list is complete hold the paper to your heart, cry onto it if necessary and resolve to let go. Then take the paper to a fireplace or outdoor space and very safely burn it. Let go. This is just one ending amongst many that create beginnings. Let your hope soar high as you make this committed clearing and offering to yourself and the soul within.

Creative Practice:
Letter to Your Pre-Pregnant Self

Cast your mind back to who you were at week one, as your period began and you were, for all intents and purposes, not pregnant. Who was that woman, and how might she be viewing the person you are today: someone who knows she is pregnant? It is likely that it feels you have leapt great canyons since then.

I therefore ask you to gently explore this, and to do so via a letter to yourself. Written from the you of now, to the you of week one. I encourage you to explain what has happened: the ups and downs you have moved through from week one to the present moment, to offer guidance, love and hand-holding. Reflect gently on all that has unfolded since the first day of that last period and share your heart with yourself. Trust that in that unfolding, that release, you help to unburden the parts of you that feel fear and help cement understandings that you may not have fully actualised, until now.

Journal Prompts

- How do I honestly feel right now?

- What do I feel most hopeful about?

- What clues did I receive in the early days of this pregnancy, and did I listen?

- What are the best and worst things about the release and letting go I am currently living through?

Affirmation: *I release all things that stand in the way of this journey.*

Week 5
Little Signs

Around week five your standard pregnancy books might say you are starting to experience the smallest of inklings that you are pregnant. The most obvious being that your period has not yet arrived. Other signs may be sore breasts, tiredness and nausea.

As you think back on your early days of pregnancy, ask yourself: *what parts of me were aware, if any, that I was pregnant?*

- Was your gut and intuition rumbling that something was new or different?

- Did you know something had changed?

- Did you feel it in your hips, your bones, your womb?

- Were you hit with a sudden wave of unexplained nausea?

- Did you feel different without explanation?

- Did you have a dream or see a sign?

- Or were you oblivious to the thickening of the womb, the subtle pangs of tender breasts, or the whispering of change within?

Writing this in my third pregnancy I can say that this time round I should have been suspicious but I put all the arising evidence down to a bad bout of sickness suffered over Christmas. My first pregnancy however, I knew about right away. I felt the egg implant into my womb whilst in my grandmother's house. There were other signs too. My father and I whispered conspiratorially over tarot cards showing women holding eggs with babies within them. My blow-up bed deflated in the night (no state of comfort for a newly pregnant woman). And I knew then. That same grandmother passed days before this third child made themselves known. Eventually when my period had been MIA for long enough, I became curious and took a pregnancy test. In this space of love and loss, familial ups and downs and some rumbling marital discontent, a child started to form.

The signs we are exploring in this chapter are not the physical symptoms of pregnancy that most books focus on, but rather the spirited, mysterious, and divine ones. I truly believe that this initiation of pregnancy will bring a great deal to your life, and some of that sits in the arena of psychic phenomena and our intuitive ability.

Before I spook you, I ought to say that these phenomena are entirely natural. I am certain you will have had uncanny experiences in your life: strong intuitive feelings, gut instincts, maybe even rumblings of the unknown that have left you feeling intrigued. Pregnancy may bring some of these internalised talents to the surface. For the ability to connect to intuition, or even more profoundly, spiritual knowing, is an innate capacity, one that you can ignore or practice. I suggest that in this liminal pregnant space, you start to gently explore it.

One way to become familiar with the 'divine' that is all around us, is through connecting to the signs that pop up in your everyday world. Being open and welcoming to such signs is powerful and will cause you to feel beautifully connected to something 'more'.

My pregnancies have always taken me deeply inside myself, but also outward, to nature and to connecting with all that surrounds me. Signs have arisen for me in a bounty of ways throughout my pregnancies. Most recently I had a worrying blood test, and when I removed the cotton wool from the injection site later that day, I noticed the blood had pooled in the form of a love heart. This felt like a sign of reassurance, one of love, from my unborn straight to me. Gross though it may be, I kept that little piece of cotton wool and referred to it whenever I was anxious about the test results! I am happy to report that the love heart was a good omen and the test came back clear.

You will also find signs arising through nature. The appearance of certain animals, or birds making a nest can feel beautifully connected to the actions you are taking to feather your own nest. You might overhear empowering words or have a conversation that hits every chord in your heart at just the right moment, leaving you feeling vibrant and alive. Maybe you dream about a beloved lost friend or relative, as you close your eyes their face pops up, and whilst you could write it off as imagination and hormones, you may also choose to see it as a loving direct contact.

Little signs are with you daily, and the magic is in allowing yourself to recognise them and experience them. This week we will be working on delving past the physical symptoms of early pregnancy and starting to dive into the spiritual ones instead.

Meditation: *Signs*

The purpose of this meditation is to meet with a meaningful 'sign' of some kind. Begin by placing one hand to your heart, and one over your womb. Take three lovely deep breaths. Imagine your energies dropping into your heart, your womb, your warm inner self. If any anxiety or stress makes itself known, imagine breathing purposefully into this space, feeling the breath begin to carry it away.

Allow your imagination to drift to a beautiful space in nature, real or imaginary, – your favourite beach, a welcoming woodland or a lush meadow. Be at one with the space you find yourself in. Surrender to rest and trust that a sign will arise in your imagination, be it a creature, an object, a word, a song, a lyric or some other meaningful interaction.

Allow your sign to arise by itself, and do not second guess it when it arrives. Try not to dismiss what emerges as too silly or random. Whatever symbol, creature or item is received, know that it is for you, and that it holds meaning that is either clear and apparent, or that will arise for you over time. Sit with this for a few minutes, allowing any thoughts, feeling or insight to bubble up.

When you have witnessed your sign, take it to heart. Trust that it holds meaning and affirmation. Stay in meditation until you feel the energies subsiding and you are ready to return to the room. Take a few deep breaths to re-energise.

Write down your sign, perhaps research it and consider what might it mean to you.

Soulful Practice:
Ask for a Sign
(and believe it when it comes)

You have received a sign in meditation, which hopefully was a gentle and easy experience. Your challenge now is to ask for one in your everyday life, and to let it find you. This is a task I have done hundreds of times over the years with many different clients and it never disappoints. Many of my clients, myself included, have experienced surprisingly wonderful cosmic affirmation because of simply asking.

Your soulful prompt is to take a few minutes to yourself, and to ask the divine/universe:

"Please give me a sign of affirmation and support for me to reflect upon within this pregnancy."

Or you may wish to be a little more specific and choose a particular sign to receive (the more random the better).

"Please give me the following sign, a XXXX as loving proof of spiritual guidance and support in this time."

Either way of asking for a sign works.

I recently asked for a sign in the form of a kite, and had all but given up when I drove past a huge factory with 'Kite' – both the word and a huge image of a kite – emblazoned in green down the very large warehouse wall. At other times I have asked for a general 'sign' and been given something profound at a meaningful moment that really felt like the universe reaching out and offering comfort.

I cannot say anything further on how this might arise for fear of ruining your personal experience or giving you expectations that stop you seeing the unique nature of your own sign. I am certain however that if you pay attention, you will be given potentially more than one sign and that what does arrive will be clear cut and beyond dispute. Try to believe the sign as it arises, you don't need anybody else's opinion, agreement or permission. This is yours, let it be yours, allow this moment of magic to be yours.

Your sign could arrive in many forms, but it will feel, for a moment, like the divine/universe/great mystery is lining up and speaking to you. It will be surprisingly easy for you to dismiss what occurs, so the real challenge is in choosing to believe. In accepting your sign, you make space for more signs to come. From here you may find similar signs repeat throughout pregnancy, or whenever you need a boost or reminder of your connection. Keep your heart and mind open! And whenever a sign appears, be sure to write it down in your journal.

 ## Creative Practice: *Vision Board*

This week's creative activity is to make a vision board filled with images of things you consider to be powerful signs and symbols – these may include ones you have received in the past, the signs that you knew you were pregnant, the signs you have asked for in the Soulful Practice or received in the Meditation.

A vision board requires magazines or printed images that you can cut up, scissors and glue and a large sheet of paper to sick them onto. You may also wish to draw some of these signs or words by hand, to bring an extra touch and personal invocation to the board.

Leaf through the images and papers you have, cutting out those things that align, be they images or words. Stick them to the page in a way that feels attractive. Continue until your page is full. This is your vision board. Keep it somewhere that you can revisit and admire. This will help provoke the manifestation of the energies upon the board but will also reconnect you repeatedly to the highest hopes of your intuitive self.

Leave space for this vision board to grow. Revisit it throughout your pregnancy, adding on new signs and symbols that occur.

 ## Journal Prompts

- How would I describe my spiritual beliefs?
- Do I believe in 'something more' and how would I define it?
- Where in the world, or in my life do I feel most 'connected' to some kind of source/power/magic that goes beyond myself? How would I describe this?
- What 'out of the ordinary' events have I experienced in my lifetime?
- Do I tend to naturally accept the spiritual or supernatural? Am I curious or sceptical and dismissive of them?

 Affirmation: *I am lovingly connected to all that is. I find peace, support and love in this connection.*

Week 6
Womb Magic

Before your pregnancy had you spent much time thinking about your womb, or indeed any organ of your body? Out of sight, out of mind, tends to be many people's approaches until such time as your body calls for attention. Usually, such cries are due to things going wrong: a dodgy kidney, a fatty liver, a palpitating heart... It is rare that we give our innards much love, other than perhaps attempts to guard and protect them via diet and lifestyle changes.

Similarly, your womb may not have come to mind too much unless it was giving you trouble. Period pains or more serious aspects of womb health may have arisen for you, causing you to see that part of the body as an occasional area of difficulty. Yet those symptoms and disruptions pale into insignificance as your womb takes on its life's work: hosting a child. It's only now you might begin to recognise the miracle and magic that has been embedded in your hip girdle all this time!

This week we will focus on celebrating the womb. No matter your relationship to this life-giving organ, no matter what hardships it may have visited on you previously, right now, it is the sanctum, the sacred host for your growing beloved. It's the safest and only place where your child might perfectly grow from tiny seed to full-term infant. So, celebration it is! Let's spend the week in reverence of this incredible life-giving space that, until now, we have may have underrated and overlooked.

 ## Meditation: *Womb Blessing*

I learned meditation and healing as a child and have always found these powers extremely easy to access. I'd like to offer this to you here and now, and for you to work with your womb to bless and heal the space. However, you may also go on to use this very simple technique on any part of your body that you wish, and indeed on pets, children, and friends. This energy is a gift, and is not as complex as something like reiki, so please do share this freely and without a need for financial compensation.

Bringing yourself to rest. Closing your eyes and begin connecting to your breath.

Imagine a bubble of white light surrounding you, keeping you safe. Feel your feet on the ground and imagine roots connecting from your feet all the way to the earth, this is to keep you grounded, connected and centred. Ask mentally or aloud that you are protected and that only the very highest energies for you and your baby's best benefit are allowed to enter this blessing.

Allow the white light within the bubble to enter your body, through your breath and perhaps through the crown chakra – a sacred space at the top of your head – or just above it. Imagine pulling this energy inwards and letting it swirl around your body, working magic.

The light begins to build up in your gut, your stomach and chest cavity, wherever feels good. You are now able to imagine the light travelling from this spiralling mass within you, down your arms and being channelled out through your hands. Place your hands on your womb and allow a channel of this healing and empowering energy to move through you and bless your womb. You may wish to say the following words or something similar:

"I welcome loving healing energetic light to my womb space. I honour my womb and the life growing within. I trust this blessing light to enable growth, safety and onward progression for myself and the babe within."

Sit with this energy until it feels like it is ebbing away. Take a moment to thank the healing blessed energy and to release it. Feel your feet on the ground, let the bubble float away, take a refreshing breath and return to the room. Take a moment to drink some cool water and return to your daily experience.

 # Soulful Practice:
Connect to Your Womb

The womb is a space we can connect to ancient fertile wisdom about who we are, our desires and a deeper level of intuition. We hear often about 'gut' instinct, and yet the womb, a place of true growth and power is another organ, much like the heart, brain or solar plexus that stores energy, memories, knowing, and infallible personal truth. In this week's practice I suggest easy daily undertakings that you can do to forge a relationship with your womb and start to hear the messages and power she contains for you.

- Take a deep breath, hands covering your womb, take a moment to connect to this space, write about anything that comes up or how you feel. Repeat this throughout the week and see what arises from your womb to your heart and mind.

- Read a book that focuses on women's wisdom and sacred power holding. Get to know the voices that are out in the world that reflect and share the wonder of the womb space beyond the biological and ordinary. You might like to explore the books *Moon Time* by Lucy H. Pearce or *Cycles of Belonging* by Stella Tomlinson.

- If you have a deck of oracle cards, it would be lovely to pull a card as a message from your womb. This space holds much wisdom, and many women connect to their wombs as their intuitive and spiritual centre.

- You could source a womb blessing from a local trusted healer or ask your usual alternative therapist what they might offer in terms of womb healing and connection. You may be surprised what is available and how powerful it is.

 Creative Practice: *Create Your Womb*

Have you ever considered your womb to be a sacred inner creative space and sanctuary? You may have seen some beautiful works of art where artists have created reflections of the womb in paint, flowers, or pencil. No matter how artistic you might feel yourself to be, this is a lovely exercise for you to replicate.

- You may simply like to gather some flowers and leaves and create a floral replication of your womb using them. This can be photographed, glued down or simply swept aside afterwards.

- You may wish to use chalk, paint or pencils to sketch out a version of your womb, perhaps with your foetus within, tucked up with hearts, flowers or whatever takes your fancy.

- Paint or colour an egg. The egg is symbolic of the cosmic space from which life hatches. You can pop a tiny hole either side of the top and bottom of the egg and blow out the innards to prevent it going rotten, then decorate the egg as you feel compelled. Add it to an altar or shelf to symbolically engage with your womb each time you notice it.

- For those who find art and drawing unappealing, you may prefer to sketch out your womb in words and poetry, perhaps using another medium such as clay, sand or rocks to mould or sculpt an image of swirling ovaries, or knitting or felt to create a beautiful fabric uterus.

The very act of engaging with your womb in this way is empowering, unexpected and fun! It may also feel rather rebellious, with the womb usually being a very tucked away and whispered part of the anatomy in our masculine-dominant culture. Reclaim your womb externally and allow this very important part of your journey to be seen and understood, even if only by your loving eyes!

Bringing the image of your womb into the outer world is a sweet exercise in reminding ourselves of the guts and glory of what is taking place within. It helps connect you to this spring of life within and bows to its almighty creativity.

 # Journal Prompts

- Take a moment to envision yourself in the womb, as you would have been at some time. What arises for you? Is it a good experience – or not? Consider how you might recreate a space of love and safety for the child within.
- Sit with the idea of your womb for a few moments, allow words, colours, symbols to bubble up. What is your womb communicating to you right now?
- What has my relationship with my womb been like in my life thus far?
- How might I kindle and foster an understanding of this space as sacred, safe, creative, wise and loving?

 Affirmation: *I trust my womb.*
I send love to my womb. My womb is my miracle.

Week 7
Fertility Rites

In our culture we tend not to talk about or focus much on fertility...unless there is an issue with it. We are either encouraged to prevent conception...or are seeking support for infertility. Otherwise, we just take fertility – our own and that of the land and other animals – for granted. But in many human cultures, fertility – asking the gods for it to be bestowed or thanking them for its fruits – is done in ritualistic and ceremonial ways as a central part of community life.

Whether becoming pregnant happened easily for you or was more of a challenge, our fertility – the ability to conceive and carry life – is to be held sacred, to be recognised for the miracle it is. As you start to see and feel the baby within grow it is powerful to think on the idea of fertility. This week our focus is on the life force that is expanding within, this may be your baby, but equally it may be aspects of yourself. Together you spiral and grow into something so much more than what you were before. For it is not just a child we are creating, but a shift in who we are, and a dance with the possibilities that this new life may bring.

Fertility can be a hard circumstance to contain and hold. Being in a continually fertile state for nine months, constantly making room for another human, will push, pull and challenge your resilience in unexpected ways. Whilst on the surface you may wear it with ease and grace and wonderful moments, the weight of fertility, of rebirthing humanity, and the lack of support for this role in our culture, may pull at your loins, heart and mind.

I believe, therefore, that some time connecting to the concept of fertility and viewing it as a rite of passage that requires reverence, will help you connect to the sacred magnitude of the task at hand.

Meditation: *The Corn Dance*

In many cultures fertility is summoned through music and dance. In England this was done by dancing around the Maypole on May Day. I was inspired to create a 'corn dance' meditation, to help celebrate the sustenance and persistence of fertility. This meditation was inspired by a card of the same name within the *Medicine Woman* tarot card deck, a beautiful array of images focused on Indigenous American imagery. I had also recently spent time in Kentucky, my mother's ancestral home, just before this pregnancy arrived. I had spent time walking around corn fields with my small family, the vibrance and energy of the corn as representative of fertility, felt deeply alive in me. My memories of playing as a child within my grandmother's vegetable patch and her lines and lines of corn bring me deep into a feeling of harvest and abundance. This meditation arose from within these combined factors...

Source some ritual music, this may be different things for different people: acapella singing, drums, or folk music. Perhaps you may feel called to classical or something traditional to a specific culture that feels appropriate. Ensure the music has a flow and won't interrupt your meditative journey.

Take a breath, get comfortable and find yourself relaxing into your body in a peaceful place.

Take your mind's eye to a meadow, in the distance you can hear the music along with joyful singing and cheers. You follow the music through the meadow, to a line of trees up ahead. You know that when you walk through the trees you will be with the people celebrating.

Walk through the trees and find yourself in a space with a fire, dancing women, children playing, and food being eaten and shared in celebration. You feel at home. You are called into the dance, and liberated from any self-consciousness, you begin to move your body to the music with the others who are moving around the fire.

You notice that you are surrounded by the abundance of fertility: fruit, corn, wheat and any other items that represent fertility to you. You are passed an ear of corn, and you recognise that this is only given to those who are wielding fertility, who are bearing a babe in their wombs. The corn is your permission to dance wildly, to honour the life being created and to recognise yourself as the vital halfway home for the soul being birthed.

Dancing around the fire, you feel deeply connected and held by the community. You are recognised as a great part in a long story. Dance till your soul is content.

When you feel ready and complete, tuck the corn into your heart or your pocket. Wave goodbye to your community and return to your meadow, from here, taking a few deep breaths and reconnecting to the moment, you may return to your daily life.

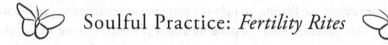

Soulful Practice: *Fertility Rites*

This week is about celebrating fertility, both your own fertility and that of the world around you. If you are not aware of the fertility rites from your own culture you may want to explore these this week, as well as those from other cultures. This does not necessarily mean the modern culture you were raised in, look further back, you may feel drawn to a particular ancient rite or way of wisdom that pre-dates the circumstances you were raised in.

Your research may involve speaking to elders, reading an empowering and informative book, or a simple Google search.

Do what you can to bring the information that you learn into your daily life. Perhaps you will feel called to visit an ancient site that is linked with fertility, or to attend a temple or church to light a candle or pray in honour of yourself and your growing child. You may choose to sit in a meadow, woodland or stone circle and gift yourself a moment to connect to the sacred within and without and marvel at the never-ending fertility of our beautiful planet.

Creative Practice: *Celebrating Fertility*

This week's Creative Practice is all about celebrating fertility. Based on your research you may wish to:

- Cross-stitch, paint or knit a fertility symbol or deity connected to fertility.
- Relish the creative joy of new life: visit a friend's new puppy, watch cute kitten videos online, find a caterpillar or some frogspawn if the season (and the law) allows and nurture it.
- Get a pot of earth and plant some seeds, water them and watch them grow from tiny shoots to mighty plants.

- Go for a walk and notice what season it is and what is growing and thriving now. Take some photographs of the fertility you witness around you.

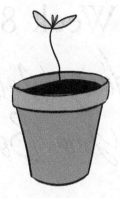

Journal Prompts

- As I move forwards in my pregnancy, what has changed, grown, and transformed within me so far?
- How can I honour the ebb and flow of my fertile energy at this time?
- As a rite of passage my pregnancy, so far, has provided great insight into the following...
- What are my sacred and spiritual intentions for this pregnancy?

 Affirmation: *I am life, I create life,*
I surrender to life.

Week 8

Finding Yourself in Your Body

A pregnancy may feel like a diamond dropped from heaven into your womb, or at times, like a war-mongering little alien has hosted itself in you determined to exhaust and sicken you. There are days that these two forces exchange themselves, with the wonder of it all swiftly replaced by a bout of nausea, the magnificence of life creation swapped out for a desperately early bedtime and avoidance of all but one food source.

Whatever experience you are currently transiting through, it is likely that it feels very different to the ordinary, everyday certainty of being yourself. Rather than seeing this as an interruption to the norm, I invite you to see your pregnancy as an opportunity to expand, not least widthways, but also, to allow your body, to have her own experience. You may have kept her locked up tight, as per the demands of society for many years with exercise and varieties of healthy (and less healthy) eating. Or you may have totally ignored the needs of your physical body with disordered eating, diets, drugs, self-harm, a lack of care... Pregnancy is an opportunity to start afresh and develop a new relationship with your body.

Pregnancy may give you a new motivation to take care of yourself: to listen to your body's needs and heed them, creating healthy habits. It may give you permission to just let your body 'be' for the first time, to ride the waves of what your body brings, to hand your body the reins and trust her to know what to do.

Our bodies are wise, they hold within them a lifetime of wisdom and an ancient instinct primed to nurture life and give birth. Remember that you carry within you the knowing of the stars. Every element of your body has been formed and reformed time and time again over the course of life on Earth, and likely before that. Trust that your body, and her celestial make up, knows what it is doing.

Our modern age of medicine and high physical standards has exacted vast demands upon our energies. Our greatest minds have added to our resilience and provided for longer lifespans, better quality of life and myriad cures. Yet still, even despite these advances and medical powers, our bodies know so much more than our conscious minds do.

As we move into this week, I want you to work on trusting the ancient wisdom of your physicality. Not fighting or judging it, but rather, giving over to it. Find yourself in your body, breathe into your core, and find comfort in the fact that your vessel, ancient and wise, knows exactly what it is doing. Even if that knowledge is strange for your mind, or hard on your gut, it is an experience of great wisdom and evolutionary magic playing itself out through you. Lucky you! Behold the priestess within and breathe deeply, trusting that all that occurs is exactly as some greater natural force has decreed.

 ## Meditation: *Body and Breath*

This week's meditation requires you to drop into your body, to listen to her needs and ponder them with respect and a desire to fulfil all that is being asked.

Play some peaceful inspiring music and get comfortable.

Breathe in and out deeply and slowly. Connect your feet to the earth (outdoors and barefoot if possible), whilst imagining your heart and head opening and connecting to the sky. Let nature's rhythm move through you. Breathe into a new speed, a new tempo. Let that tempo be one that finds you. Let it carry you. Let the breath be a new composition, one that releases you from any chains you have placed on your physical self. As you find the rhythm allow your muscles to let go of whatever they might be holding, and give permission for your cells to surrender to a new peacefulness.

Repeat this several times throughout the week. Let your body lead. Let the breath become circular and powerful. See these moments of deep breathing as moments of disconnecting the chains of the mind and movement into innate natural wisdom. Become aware of your vibrations, your tiny motions, the flicks of your eye and loosening of muscles. Be in a closeness with your being and let that pull your life forward.

Soulful Practice:
Breathe. Eat. Rest. Trust.

Allow yourself to begin to trust that you don't need to do anything. Your hair grows, your injuries heal themselves, your heart beats and your skin rejuvenates over and over to keep you tied up in a neat little human package. Your baby becomes itself without you lifting a finger. This week we move into a place of trust and surrender. We release ourselves to the hope, love and grace of the forces within us that have no voice, but that conjure our existence over and over again.

Your Soulful Practice is to purposefully provide for your body. Be acutely aware of what your physical self is asking for, and provide it: a walk, a glass of water, several deep breaths, an early night… Let your body speak her needs, and you, in reverence and worship of her, loyally and dutifully provide them.

This could be the start of a whole new relationship with yourself. One where you release the chains of what you think ought to be done. Replacing that harsh reality with a reality of listening and obeying the deep fundamental knowing of your bones, flesh, and organs.

Creative Practice:
Create a Nature Table or Garden

Nature is wise beyond our understandings: she spirals and cycles in ways that reflect our own natural wisdom. In honour of the nature working within you our creative task is to bring nature closer, to observe her, and to create some form of space or altar to her within our homes or gardens.

Gather items that you already own, or that you have close by (found on a walk or in your outdoor space) and start to form a small collection of wonder to observe and be with. You can create this as a sacred space, a place to meditate or an altar upon which you remember your own innate wilderness. I would recommend that your nature table contains all kinds of found and foraged elements of the earth. If we explore the four elements, you may wish to include:

Air – feathers, incense, fallen leaves.

Earth – pebbles, crystals, flowers, fruit, vegetables, a seedling sown in a small pot, a houseplant.

Water – a seashell, a cup of water, dew collected early in the morning in a small receptacle.

Fire – a candle, oil burner, some ash, sage, charcoal or other herbs to be burned safely.

Alongside this ode to the elements, you might include your own special memories and connections to nature: a photo of yourself in the wild, a necklace or personal item that brings you to yourself, a bunch of wildflowers you collected.

This altar or natural space is one that will serve you through pregnancy. It can be refreshed as the mood takes you and the seasons shift. Visit it regularly and place your hopes and intents upon it. Allow loved ones to add their magic and hope. Let this space become an ode to the life you are creating both deeply within your womb, and the life that transforms within your own understandings of who and what you are.

Journal Prompts

- What is my body saying right now?

- How have I kept my body's needs on a tight leash?

- As I begin to listen to the needs of my physical self, I notice the following requests and patterns...

- Take three, long, slow breaths, tune into your body. What changes? How does the release of breath allow for a settling and relaxation that feels very different?

Affirmation: *I trust my body to lead the way.*

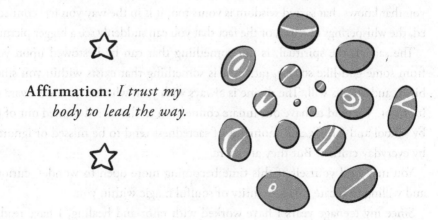

Week 9
Heightened Spirituality

Pregnancy is a time of heightened connection to a spiritual path. If I have not made that clear throughout previous weeks, then I am stating it more clearly now. Pregnancy is an initiation to our inner experience of the world, which fully includes our experience of our divine spark. The divine is deeply present in all of life and can be found in every gritty interactive moment. In pregnancy, in the growing and nurturing of another human soul, we become a hot house of intuition, magical knowing and a desire for the sacred.

You may find yourself lusting for that elusive connection to spirit, something to help you feel buoyed up and held. Pregnancy is transformative, and yet, unless your partner or friends have grown a baby themselves, their perspective and support may at times feel lacking or partial. They may be completely unaware of the incredible spiritual aspects of the journey. You may find yourself wishing to lean on something more magical than a hand hold or a backrub. I promise you that this connection is already forged, and this week we will find ways to better explore it.

Conventionally it is shown that the man at the front of the temple or the church is the only one holding sacred wisdom and connection. Yet, there is something in you that knows that sacred wisdom is yours too. It is in the way you feel connected, the whisperings of truth, or the fact that you can suddenly see a bigger picture.

The sacred, the spiritual, is not something that can be bestowed upon you from some god-like source, rather, it is something that exists within you since birth, and always will. The divine is always with you, whether you are aware of it or not. We tend to have our innate connection to the sacred trained out of us by school and family, and moments of sacredness tend to be missed or ignored by everyday culture. But they are there.

You may find yourself at this time becoming more open to wonder, curious and willing to locate this lost entity of soulful magic within you.

Since my teenage years I have worked with tarot and healing, I have read a thousand spiritual books on all kinds of subjects and immersed myself in alternative faiths, meditation and interesting practices. What I always come back to is this: the sacred is with me now, in its most beautiful raw forms and it is best experienced through all my relationships, the grit of life, my overcoming of difficult situations, the way nature shows up to meet me. As I became a mother and a parent, it infiltrated that too, the honour and sacrifice and surrender that this time of life requires is the fastest path to spiritual understanding I've ever had the intensity and pleasure to experience!

Whether you have had a life packed with spiritual experiences or this is a whole new dimension you are just starting to explore, this book will help to nudge the soulful to the surface. The key is to allow it. To let pregnancy be the prompt you need to stop and pay attention. To begin to see the patterns in your life. To observe how one thing leads to another. This is the perfect time to conjure your experiences with the magical unknown and choose to believe in them. Witness your own unexpected wisdom. Feel that connection that begs to be acknowledged. Notice the synchronicity that brought you to certain people and situations. Let that intuition be heard. Trust that the rainbow or the robin or the smell of your grandma's perfume materialising is something tangible and meaningful. Spirituality requires trust in that which lies beyond what the eye can see, trust beyond that which the mind can know. Trust your own intuition and senses and let them be the new guide to your everyday.

This week I ask you to give over to this trust and start to see your life through the lens of sacred possibility.

 # Meditation: *Calling in the Spiritual*

This meditation acts as a bridge between yourself and your spiritual aspects, helping them to unite on your pregnancy journey. This can help heighten your connection and awareness to self, the divine and the wider world.

Bring yourself into a relaxed state, taking a few deep breaths and allowing the day to drift away as you sit or lie in a relaxed posture. Give yourself to this moment and imagine any problems or anxieties dropping away, leaving you with a clear space. You might imagine your mind becoming flooded with a relaxing colour, grounding yourself and giving yourself permission to rest and stop here for a while...

As you move into fuller relaxation take a moment to begin to visualise, doing so in whatever way connects easily to you, this may be through mental imagery, imaginative picturing or something different such as sound, listening, bodily feelings etc.

Imagine you are taking a walk along a path that feels familiar and known. You are safe and all around you are fields and open expanses of great beauty. Take some time to meander down the path, headed to a space, known and yet unknown, familiar and yet new.

Allow your meandering to take you to a bridge crossing over a gentle river. On the other side of the bridge is the spiritual world, the divine, the beauty of some great wonderful other... Gaze across and notice anything that springs to your eye. Does it look like our earthly plane, or is it quite different in shapes, colour, texture and sounds?

When you are ready begin to take a few steps towards the middle of the bridge, you are not going to cross completely, to do so is not for now and would be impossible. You are simply broaching the divide between your human parts and your divine parts. As you walk towards the middle of the bridge, you might wish to call in your spiritual 'team', any guides, helpers or gods that you are aware of, and/or if this is new, simply state the following.

"I ask the loving and supportive divine to meet me here, I call in aspects of my spiritual life that are for my highest good and greatest wellbeing."

Stand still and wait. Allow a flow of connection to find you, remain open minded about how the spiritual shows up to meet with you. Trust that a connection is being forged and that this midway meeting will serve to open you gently to a more spiritual aspect of your life. Stay with this connection until such time as it starts to ebb away.

When the moment feels right thank the divine for bringing you this connection and start to return to your side of the bridge, walking back to the familiar path, eventually allowing the path to drift away as you return to your current day and reality.

Take an energising deep breath, stretch and yawn. Come back to your day. Make notes in your journal about how this meditation played out for you and anything particularly interesting that happened.

Soulful Practice: *Pray*

Prayer is a beautiful way to create a conscious connection to self, and indeed to any higher power you choose to believe in. This purposeful conversation is more powerful than all the half thoughts that your mind indulges every single day. Prayer is a specific and purposeful channel towards answers and peace. You do not need to pray to a god, angel or any form of deity, your prayer can simply be offered up to self, to your inner wisdom, to the sanctum of clarity within. I find that prayer helps us to be very specific in honing what we really want and creating a pathway for intriguing responses to be returned.

This week I recommend you experiment with prayer. Before bed, or a few moments when you wake are beautiful times to chat with your inner guides. This can be formal or informal, whatever works for you. Trust that in creating this communication, you are beginning to awaken any parts of your knowledge and self-trust that have become dormant. Blather away, chitter chatter or be very specific with your needs and desires. And remember to listen! Be open to the rewards it brings and the surprising answers that find their way to you.

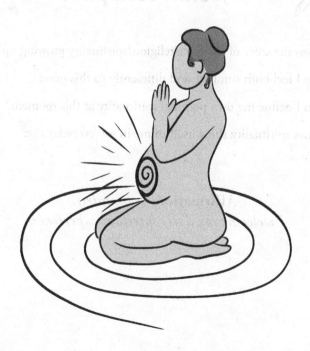

Creative Practice: *Spiritual Board*

As you connect to the bounty of your inner world this week and make space for higher possibilities and hopeful intuitive knowing, it is a powerful time to work towards those beautiful things you wish to bring into your life. A spiritual board is much like a vision board but is deeply helpful as a tool of spiritual visualisation and personal affirmation, and the act of creating your board is meditative, intuitive and magical.

A spiritual board can be a mêlée of inspiring art, passages from sacred texts, prayers, poems, sacred symbols, deities, sacred places, sacred tools... Your spiritual board is an external creation of your beliefs and your inner path: it is unique to you. By observing your spirit in this way, you bring it a step closer.

Gather glue, scissors, papers and magazines and a large sheet of paper. Begin to connect with your spiritual ideas and beliefs. Get busy with pens, paint, chalk, or dried flowers. Design this board as a direct reflection of your inner soul and allow it to reverberate your bountiful energy and longings back to you every time you witness it. This would make a very special backdrop to your altar.

Journal Prompts

- What was the story of my faith/religion/spirituality growing up?
- How do I feel both similarly and differently to this now?
- How do I define my own personal spirituality at this moment?
- How does spirituality show itself to me in my everyday life?

 Affirmation: *I am spirit.*
I welcome my daily spiritual experiences.

Week 10

Attachment and Non-Attachment

Many of us have built a life upon performance: performing for our parents, teachers, friends and employers. Pregnancy and the life to come ushers in a new powerful reign of self-awareness. As we move towards birthing and parenting a child, so we must move closer to our inner truth, the version of us that we were always meant to be. This path induces a shedding and letting go of the masks and performances we have worn, so that we can become an authentic version of self.

The more we focus on releasing who we were and how we thought our future might be, the more we recognise how much we have become attached to people, places and things (and of course ideas, hopes and ambitions), as well as different versions of ourselves.

Buddhists and many other people of faith actively work towards 'non-attachment' in their lives, reckoning that in doing so, they are freed from the everyday painful feelings many of us experience. This always felt a little problematic to me when it comes to parenting. As parents (or future parents) our children's survival and emotional wellbeing is doubtless dependent upon our attachment to them.

As a mother who has joyfully undertaken an attachment style of parenting, I am always aware of the deep need for physical and emotional closeness in parenting. Indeed, attachment is where we are right now, literally and physically, our baby is attached, through implantation, and later by the umbilical cord to the placenta to us. Attachment to our child, to their needs, is fully acceptable and beautifully warranted.

I do, however, believe that there is something powerful to this concept of letting go that will serve ourselves and our future child. Getting the balance right, recognising where to let go, and where to hold tight, is the magic of being truly present. Presence to the moment is one of the most powerful tools of wellbeing and soulfulness that life can offer us. To best service your attachment to your unborn child, and your personal growth, you may find a growing need to detach from certain people, places and things that do not serve you. There is work to be done, and undone here, it takes energy and inner reserves, and yet, the attachment we are working towards is one that is life affirming, and indeed, life creating.

The path to personal sovereignty is one littered with that which did not and does not work. To become a parent is to enact a spiritual pilgrimage, not to some far-flung temple, but to the temple within. The closer you can get to your truth, the more comfortable you will be in your parental skin. This week we will focus on nurturing healthy attachment and purposeful letting go of unhealthy or old attachments.

The purpose of this week's practices is to create a more genuine base of stability from which to move forward into the depths of your pregnancy. Your energy may be higher and more visceral than usual, your hopes and dreams more potent and alive. This is a good time, within the early stages of pregnancy, to begin the journey to figure out who you are. Really, truly, devotedly, who you are.

 # Meditation: *Releasing Attachments*

Begin by placing one hand to your heart, and one over your womb. Take three lovely deep breaths. Imagine your energies dropping into your heart, your womb, your warm inner self. If any anxiety or stress makes itself known, imagine breathing purposefully into this space, feeling the breath begin to carry it away.

Within this meditation I ask you to consciously breathe, and to allow your mind to carry you towards a time and place when you felt that you were most authentically yourself. Pay attention to this memory and the feeling of it when it floats up. Do not judge what you find here. This truth of who you are may have been pushed down and told they were not good enough. Do not allow that negativity into this space. Instead focus on the raw feeling of power that being 'you' inhabited.

What did this feel like in your mind, heart, emotions and personal confidence? Let this feeling grow and expand. Do not repress or push this down. Allow yourself permission to be this moment of your greatest self. Let the flow of this energy get bigger. Be this person, in all your nooks and crannies, in all your facets and personality traits. Allow this truth to become the totality of you.

Now let yourself notice the things that pull you from this truth of who you are: habits, emotions, memories, people, roles… All of these are attachments that stand in the way and interrupt the purest version of who you really are.

Imagine them like thorns that have pierced themselves to your skin or clothes as you have walked through life. Witness each one with love and compassion. Imagine taking it in your hands and unhooking it gently, naming it aloud and saying, " [...] I release you."

Let anything that stands in the way of your true self be shed like old skin. There is no space for any doubt or inner conflict, imagine it all dropping off. Visualise yourself becoming bigger and more profound than the version of you that you have inhabited to quell and calm others. Become your shiniest, boldest self.

Taking a long breath imagine anchoring and embedding this truth of yourself into your heart and mind. Repeat three times...

"I release all old attachments. I give myself permission to be fully me."

Breathe and sit till any big feelings subside. Shake off any remnants of doubt or pain that wish you to be anything other than yourself. Taking a beautiful full breath, return to the room.

You may wish to write in your journal about the attachments that emerged for you and how releasing them makes you feel. Record in writing the version of yourself that you witnessed and think about where that person sits within you now and why they may not have been prominent.

 ## Soulful Practice: *An Altar to You!*

Create a little altar dedicated to yourself. This is a space that you fill with aspects of you – all your positive and life affirming attachments. Perhaps a childhood photo, your most beloved piece of jewellery, a shell you picked up on a beach, a flower or plant you most love. Light a candle and gaze upon this shrine that represents the heart of you!

Take a moment to honour all that you are, and all that you have the potential to become. As you sit with this moment it is a good time to speak to your own inner self, and trust that the depleted and repressed parts of you are listening. This is a deeply intimate moment with you, just as you are, separate from any other being, be they child or beloved. What kindness and love will you offer yourself, without apology, excuse or permission?

Create a list focused on your precious attachments to yourself: loving acts you might offer to your own being. Keep this in your sight over the coming weeks with a devotion to self becoming a top priority.

Creative Practice: *A Self-Portrait*

Whatever your art skills, this is a fun task. You may doodle, sketch, photograph or watercolour your way to this piece of artwork. What matters most about this self-portrait is that it is a representation of yourself as you and you alone.

The purpose of this week's creation is to capture your unique spark. You may write around your image, or underneath it, descriptions of all that is exquisitely yours. Big yourself up. You are the vessel that contains someone else (and will be forever attached), and it must be adored, worshipped and found to be so very worthy. Focus on those aspects of yourself that you wish to remain true forever: the glory and the glow, the magic and the mastery.

This artistic version of you will perhaps be inspired by the vision of your best most truthful self you met within your meditation. Even if it feels a far cry from where you are day-to-day, this is a semblance of something within: a part of you wanting to expand and evolve and take up more space. Let your light and magic shine through the page, even if just in scribbled words and swirly representations.

Journal Prompts

Take a moment to journal about all the areas in life where you share your energy. These may be places such as work, helping aging parents, assisting your partner, domestic chores, caring for other children, friends…

- How have some of these attachments come to define me?

- How can I let go of attachments that are draining or no longer serving me?

- How might some of this energy be reclaimed? What would I like to use it for instead?

- Where and with whom do I feel safest to be my truest and most vulnerable self?

- Create a list of things you are letting go of and saying no to.

 Affirmation: *I let go of anything that stands*
between myself and my most beautiful truth.

Week 11
Navigating Chaos

Pregnancy has the potential to be chaotic. It brings lots of situations to the surface that require our attention. This can feel tumultuous, as life appears to throw problem after problem our way, and yet choosing to deal with this proactively can be tremendously healing and surprisingly helpful.

I have found my current pregnancy to be a hot bed of things problematic: if it's not one thing, it's been something else. Much of it has felt very much outside of my control. I have had to centre myself within what has felt like an onslaught of happenings, to try to get the best view, to watch what is occurring, and to calmly elevate myself into practical, loving and helpful responses. I have repeatedly chosen to be with **this** moment, rather than avoiding it. This approach has led to some surprising personal growth and the creation of space for others to do their personal growing within too.

Often one of the most powerful routes we can take to overcome difficulty in life is to choose to actively experience the circumstances we are in. It can be tempting to freeze or run away from stressful situations, but sometimes the hardships of life require our attention for them to be surmounted. This week I will encourage you to bring yourself to the moment fully. You will choose to witness and observe what is happening and to dive deeply into how that makes you feel, and what you are willing to do about it. This approach does not mean you should react, but rather, you are to 'be' in the moment, and objectively observe and witness events as they unfold.

Whatever difficulties raise their heads throughout this time are for you to scrutinise and to feel your way around. Standing back, taking an objective stance and perhaps seeing what there is to address, change or learn from, can be just the medicine to help you cultivate the clarity that you desperately need in the midst of chaos. Try to elevate your perspective slightly, and certainly allow others to resolve their own difficulties where they can. Take on only what is necessary, and be present to sit calmly with the rest of life, this will allow for you to have heightened and evolved responses and reactions.

In working with my own spiritual path and supporting many others on theirs, I have over time come to see that often difficulty helps to cause the change we sorely need. Whilst hard circumstances can feel deeply unpleasant, they do come loaded with possibility and gifts. This eventful time of growing a child is liable to raise more than your usual share of bizarre and challenging events. Trust that in time this creates pathways and passageways to new understandings. As situations arise, find yourself considering what message or opening it may be providing for you to shift, grow, heal or create real life change. View and live through your drama differently, and watch as your personal growth and understandings rapidly advance.

This week I invite you to experience the chaos in your life with curiosity and with half a mind to allowing what it brings. With babe in belly (and later in arms) this is a truly helpful approach to take. For the path you are choosing – to give life – is one shot through with bounty, beauty and the bizarre. Connecting to the magic of all these things, even the challenging parts, is a power move. Welcome and fully experience your chaos with trust and hope that it is taking you towards helpful growth and change.

 ## Meditation: *Blue Sky Magic*

Breathing deeply, closing your eyes, come to a state of rest.

Bring yourself inward, imagine your consciousness spiralling from the anxiety and energy of your head and settling inwardly, to a place that is buried deep within, a space of clear knowing, open blue skies and certainty. Allow your thoughts and energy to rest in this place. Perhaps envisioning a beach or meadow, with clear sky for miles, fresh air and only the sounds of nature.

Breathe into this place of knowing and calm, letting it take your current worries and transmuting them, softening your edges and helping you to feel content and calm within your own skin. Gaze up to the blue sky with nothing to worry about, no problem to solve, a moment with your inner freedom.

Sit with this meditation as often as is necessary this week, even if only for a brief moment. A minute in the toilet cubicle at work, or before you fall asleep at night, will help bring the reality of this inward sustaining energy forward, helping you to deal wisely with all that comes your way.

Soulful Practice:
Tools for Staying in the Moment

This week allow your yourself to be fully present to whatever arises internally. Lean into the possibility that any feelings and thoughts or unexpected events are here to be worked with, witnessed and fully experienced.

Honour the importance of giving attention fully to the moment. If you feel tempted to switch off or shift into dissociation, pull yourself to the events at hand. Do what you can to connect with what is here and now. As you bring your full self to events, you allow them to be processed and to pass.

Giving your energy to the moment (without losing your sanity to it) is a healthy and constructive approach to the everyday. There is deep satisfaction in being consciously present, and working with what arises. Trust your ability to handle what comes. Here are a few suggestions to help you stay more present when your mind threatens to wander.

- You may find that you require a physical cue to help you remain in the moment. Taking a deep breath is the simplest way to remain in the here and now and can be done wherever you are, whatever the circumstances.

- Another effective and simple tool is tapping. Whenever you feel that events are whirling around you and you may get lost to your reaction or a desire to escape, try this…

  Tap gently on a bodily spot of your choice, your third eye, your wrist or your temples. Repeat the following: "I stay present, and I observe peacefully". You may wish to combine this with a few purposeful deep breaths.

- Whenever possible, make efforts to feel your feet on the floor. If you can, slip off any shoes and socks and place your bare feet to the floor. If the weather is appropriate, then do it on the grass outside.

- Focus on your immediate senses. Take a moment to notice the smells, sounds, flavours, temperature and feel of the moment. Use these as cues to remain grounded and connected to the here and now.

- Combining these physical and energetic approaches will help you stay in the moment.

Creative Practice: *Create Through Chaos*

Whilst we are bringing our attention to our lives in powerful ways, a beautiful outlet for any drama and chaos is, of course, our creativity. This week your prompt is to swirl and whirl with the unknown, to let chaos find its way through you in patterns, forms and unexpected beauty. Here are some ideas of ways you might embody all that is unruly through your art.

Splash paint around the page like a child. Chuck it at the page or pour it on and make a purposeful mess, see what happens as you layer colours without care.

Work photographically with imbalance and movement. Instead of focusing on still, posed images, bring your camera or camera phone to energetic scenarios. Spin on a chair and photograph your subject, take images from a moving vehicle, photograph in the dark whilst you or your subject dances. See how when moving into a less controllable study of the image you create surprising beauty.

Create something messy using clay. Clay for me is innately chaotic and hard to control.

Dance wildly, allow your body to discharge all its pent-up energy into movement and rhythm.

Invent a recipe or take a familiar one and give it a twist. Start from scratch and abandon your recipe book in favour of a taste and smell approach to your next meal.

Journal Prompts

- What is chaotic in my life right now? How might I wisely and calmly approach this chaotic situation this week?

- Where am I wasting energy on situations that are not mine?

- What is my usual approach to chaos (run away/freeze/ignore/dramatize etc)? What might I do this week to shift and change my conditioned response and do something different?

 Affirmation: *As I bring focus to the daily events of life, I become more empowered.*

Week 12
The In-Between

This week is an odd one. Your sap may be rising, though you are still dogged by symptoms that slow your roll. As far as the world is concerned, you probably don't look pregnant, and yet the nag at your waistband says otherwise. You may be waiting on a scan and some formal confirmation, whilst dodging your favourite food and craving the unexpected. The people who do know you are pregnant ask how you are in a deeply concerned and loving way. Whilst others carry on throwing tasks and expectations your way, and likely you bravely take up the challenges convinced you are capable, interspersed by twinges in your lower stomach muscles and an ever-present need to pee.

This is often a week fuelled by excitement, anxiety and anticipation. Many of you will have been for (or are due to attend) a scan and have the first glimpse of your new reality bubbling away within. This can feel like a real awakening, taking a concept previously only proven by a pee stick and giving it movement, a heartbeat and limbs.

It is a time of deep contradiction and shifting energies. Trust however that pregnancy is a sacred zone that is spiralling you towards some unknown future. There are times in life when the unknown feels deeply welcome and others where it is abhorrent. In pregnancy we may swerve between fear and hope, power and lack of it. At times this is disconcerting, and at other times we welcome this huge transition and the ability it carries to reframe everything. The loving way in which pregnancy takes life out of our hands can be as startling as it is deeply welcome. This will stand you in good stead for many other liminal places in pregnancy and beyond (transition during labour, the first days post birth…) the times that are neither quite this nor that, or both/and.

This time, it seems, is an 'in-between space'. You are between clothing sizes, between the knowing and unknowing of scans and doctoral confirmation, you are almost between trimesters and certainly between the anonymity of your pregnancy being secret and the inevitable announcement that comes with a growing waistline or your social media announcement that 'we are having a baby'.

As you move through this week, it's best to embrace the temporary nature of it. It is good practice for the road that lies ahead. For often with a babe in arms, it can feel like life will be like this forever. Yet the child grows quickly, and the phases that charmed or terrified you are soon lost to the mists of time. This week, with all its 'neither here nor there' energy, is fleeting. Losing ourselves to the intensity of it may be part of the trip of pregnancy, and yet, it's nice to temper that loss with a reminder that any awkwardness or flush of magic is set to give way to the next passage in your own, and your child's, growth.

This week we will focus on controlling what we can, allowing answers to come to us (rather than trying to think them up) and trusting that unknown road ahead which some days feels so close, and others so very far.

Similarly, right now you may feel as though you are spiralling a little physically, perhaps between the early phase symptoms and a surprising freedom from those symptoms. Space is being cleared, and you might consider your energy is somewhat higher. Whatever your emotional and physical feelings, this remains a strange space in which to sit. You are called to trust the contradictions and uncertainty of this moment, opening to the possibility that it is all beautifully sacrosanct and strangely perfect.

Meditation: *The In-Between Space*

Begin by placing one hand to your heart and one over your womb. Take three lovely deep breaths. Imagine your energies dropping into your heart, your womb, your warm inner self. If any anxiety or stress makes itself known, imagine breathing purposefully into this space, feeling the breath begin to carry it away.

Gently guide yourself to the in-between space you find yourself in. Perhaps you envision you are on a boat out on a lake, far from home, and yet not at your future destination. You know you can't go backwards, so you float gently, without an oar towards a future where you can envision a shining light far ahead on a sandy shore.

This space is yours. Nobody can reach you here, and it feels safe. Just as your baby lies curled within you, you sit atop the maternal waters of Mother Earth. Just as baby has no awareness of what the future holds, nor do you. And yet, you feel trust.

Trust feels and looks like an energy – what colour is it? Choose any colour that feels correct and imagine the energy of beloved conviction surrounding you and soaking your skin. It permeates your bones, your flesh, your heart and your mind. You feel trust swelling within you, with every breath it becomes you. Perhaps you notice that with this expectation of safety and hope, the sun shines a little brighter, you catch the birdsong in the distance, your boat seemingly moves a little closer to its desired destination.

Be with this as long as you like.

To remain more passive simply choose to receive the trust, let it soak into you with power and love.

If you wish the meditation to be more active, more creative, you may consider parts of your life you are ready to move beyond. Imagine throwing them overboard for the lake to transmute. Following on from this, you might choose to envision the space left by this release, and in doing so, gently contemplating what you would like to grow from here…

Stay in this space as long as you like.

When you are ready, connect to your body, take a long deep breath, visualise the boat and the lake ebbing away and return to your physical space. Take a few moments to breathe and stretch before returning to your day.

Repeat this meditation as often as needed.

 ## Soulful Practice: *The Call*

Go to bed with a specific question or call for help. There may be situations confounding you or calling for answers. As you slip into sleep each evening, do so with a purposeful intent to create clarity and solutions (whilst being willing and open to what those solutions may be). You may wish to keep your journal by the bed with the queries written in it. Keep the journal close by come morning. The answers may be sudden or take several days. They may float up during your daily doings, or in a week or two. By opening your consciousness to this call for assistance, you shift up your energy and create space for answers to arise.

Creative Practice:
Making Space for Creativity

This week is a powerful time to creatively make space. This involves the dreaded sorting through of tasks, clearing of piles and ticking off 'to-do' list scenarios. Whilst this may not feel outwardly creative, it is an invitation to creativity.

By clearing your built-up clutter, you begin to wisely prepare for the rise in your energies that is due in the weeks ahead. Meet that rising with a clear space and nothing to do. Nothing blocks and distracts from creativity quite like errands, secret piles, unopened bills, cluttered in-trays and messy drawers. Conjure the will to tackle a few things per day and feel the relief as these toxic burdens drop away and allow space for emergence.

This week you focus on freeing yourself, physically, mentally and materially, so that you can start to grow with your surroundings. Whilst you may be straddling the unknown, I encourage you to do so in your most beautiful adornments, with a cheer that grows inwardly and finds itself in the nooks and crannies of your home. Find creativity in a change of attire, a shift in routine, an invitation to those you love to be in togetherness differently. Make space and from this place feel free to see things anew and live with creativity as a calling card to possibility.

Journal Prompts

- How does being in the in-between space feel to me?
- How have I navigated the liminal before?
- How am I trying to impose certainty in this space of liminality?
- How might I rebel against my daily routine and start to insert little acts of creativity? Consider three things…

 Affirmation: *I intensify my trust.*
I trust. I am trust.

SECOND TRIMESTER

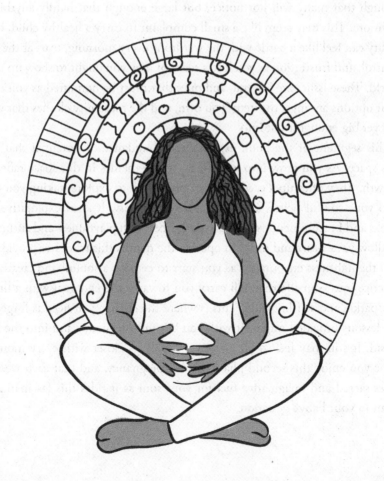

We are heading into the second trimester, a space renowned to be more energetic and connected than those early queasy days, or the later lumbering ones. There is for sure an energy of growth and expansion in this period that is quite the invitation. It calls us to motherhood and parenthood with such ferocity that at times you may forget you are pregnant. Other times, however, you might still be beholden to intriguing symptoms that remind you with a startle that you carry within you a new life. It's a funny, wonderful and weird portion of time that still has the capacity to make you vomit, whilst liberating you to take up the reins of life where perhaps you have let them go.

By week twelve your baby is fully formed in terms of limbs, parts and organs, from now on it's a journey of continued growth. You might consider the hard work is done, as hopefully the tiredness and sickness start to ebb away.

Pregnancy doubtless continues to be a time of mixed emotion. You may find yourself struggling with your changing body, particularly as any growth is subtle enough that many will not notice, but large enough that hardly anything fits anymore. This may seem like a small complaint to carry a healthy child, but the reality can feel like a battle with the wardrobe every morning, tears at the loss of control, and frustration as you lose a sense of how you ought to show up in your world. These issues are visceral, and ones that must be honoured as you explore your options amongst the items you own, and the maternity clothes that you are not yet big enough to fit into.

This segment of the book explores the abundance of potential that sits in this space. As you grow into your body, so the themes in this space reflect that growth. They offer up a cacophony of possibility to explore, taking you deeper into your soulful beliefs and your creative capacity. It is an explorative set of weeks and I recommend you take to each week with playfulness and enthusiasm.

Allow your heart and mind to open to the depths this trimester provides, but also the lightness encouraged as you start to cement a soulful and creative new practice into your life that will carry you towards the end goal with a little extra sparkle and self-knowing. This is where the change you need is forged, and the lessons provided might sit with you beyond pregnancy and into the life up ahead. It still may feel so far away, yet it gallops closer with every moment. I hope you enjoy this second phase of your pregnancy, and that each week provides sacred and imaginative fuel for your soul as it rides this fascinating moment in your baby's gestation.

Week 13
Family Tree

This week our focus will bring us outside of ourselves, using family and ancestors as a focus. It can at times feel as though we are the only one who has ever been pregnant, ever felt this way, yet a trip back into our history tells different. You are not alone in this experience; it is the act that connects you to all your ancestors, and to the family of humanity.

I remember in my first pregnancy feeling particularly anxious about giving birth. Birth had always felt a little like a threat that my femaleness carried with it, rather than a bountiful or life affirming activity of intensity and wonder that I now view it as. The one thing that I would return to when faced with the overwhelm of birth, was reminding myself that my grandmothers had done this immense same thing. That they had brought children forth from their bodies, and gone on to be healthy, interesting, quirky and beloved members of my lifetime. They had survived, thrived and gifted me love and wisdom. The 'threat' I was perceiving was something to adapt to, and the evidence that this was doable was there in the women whom I know and love.

Indeed, this thought would expand, reminding me that billions of women had birthed and raised children throughout history in circumstances akin to my own and indeed in circumstances far more or far less privileged. This connection, this good company of ancestral and modern-day birthing souls felt like wings at my back, a roar in my soul, and a reminder that birth, motherhood and parenting is another rite of passage, walked by the many, and therefore a place to stand in deep holy connection.

Creating a connection, to real, or even imagined family, is one way to bring our bodies, hearts and minds together with the task at hand. You are not alone in what is to come. You are amongst billions of birthing mothers, people and even creatures, forming a circle of infinite life and evolving with each babe to something more than you ever were before. It is overwhelming, and yet, entirely connecting.

Often it is only when we become pregnant, and our family tree starts to furl out into the future from our bellies, that we take time to look back at where and who we come from...

Now is a powerful time to spiritually connect to those in our family lines (known or unknown) and to begin thinking about the family tree we wish to create from this moment onward.

 # Meditation: *Ancestral Power*

Light a candle and play some soothing music. Find yourself in a position, such as lying down or fully supported by a sofa, where you can release and give over entirely.

Begin by placing one hand to your heart and one over your womb. Take three lovely deep breaths. Imagine your energies dropping into your heart, your womb, your warm inner self. If any anxiety or stress makes itself known, imagine breathing purposefully into this space, feeling the breath begin to carry it away.

Spend a few moments creating a visualisation in your mind of a beautiful meadow, in which stands the most astounding tree. You will recognise this tree as your own, the tree of your family and ancestors. It holds the greatest love and proudest moments of your own lineage. This need not be a history you have a huge awareness of, but trust that no matter your familial origin and circumstances, there is good, love and power within the limbs, roots and soaring branches of the tree!

Imagine yourself moving towards the tree and sitting close to it, perhaps with your back against the bark, or even climbing up into its branches and being held safely there. This is a profoundly blissful place, allow the feeling of connection and being held to flow through you.

If you feel comfortable to do so, you may wish to ask the energy of your loving and powerful ancestors to visit you. Allow this to arise however it wishes. It may be a feeling, an image, a vision, a word, a memory, a scent or some other form of knowing. Trust that this call to your ancestors is one that will echo through the coming weeks, and you may find their connections arising gently in your everyday. Allow what comes to be accepted, and to be the perfect moment of affirmation for you.

Stay with this for as long as it feels comfortable. When you are ready you may bring yourself away from the tree (knowing you can revisit whenever you desire) and return to your body, this day, your space. Take an energising breath. Wiggle, stretch and open your eyes.

Soulful Practice:
Connect with a Lost Loved One

Whatever your faith, spirituality, or lack thereof, there is much to be gained by exploring those who came before us. For some the lost loved one may spring to mind quickly and easily: a parent, grandparent, favoured aunt or family friend (it need not be a blood relative). Whether you choose to connect here on a spiritual level or simply conjure this loved one to your heart and mind, the effect is the same. You choose to remember the life that they gave you, the inspiration that guided you, the love you felt and the offering that this has for you in this moment.

Find a photograph, or if one does not exist, a totem of some kind can stand in its place (a rose for your grandma who loved roses, a button to reflect your uncle's business suits or a stone to represent the certainty of ancestors long forgotten). Make a space on a window ledge, or in a place you visit often, and create a mini shrine, a sacred place to remember, even if just for a moment each day.

If you are disconnected from family or cannot seek backwards to a soul who fulfils this role for you, feel free to choose someone from the family of your own making, a good friend, a beloved teacher or even an icon or character from a book. The essence you conjure here is important, as is the feeling this person gave to you. In reflecting on that, you heighten their good within you.

For those both with and without clear family connections, you may choose to reach back to some unknown person from your family's ancient history. You do not need to name them or know them. Understand that somebody exists from a time long before you, who was good, who you can gather comfort from, who perhaps would have empathy and compassion for you and your life. You can choose to honour this energy, alongside any other personalities or characters. You may simply create a vase of interchangeable wildflowers in their honour, naming this vase, 'the good and beloved within my line'.

Spend gentle passing time with this shrine each day. Speak your wishes and hopes to it. Ask the energies held within it for strength, hope or answers. Allow this to open a portal beyond yourself and your everyday life to the history your flesh has held, and the wonder that travels down timelines through you and onward now into your unborn.

Creative Practice: *Family Tree Tapestry*

Our practice this week is to create some form of family tree which you can keep as a keepsake for your child, or perhaps add to your altar or display in pride of place on the lounge wall.

There are so many ways you can undertake this. I will leave it to your creative peculiarities to sort through and design, but I hope you will find it an empowering and interesting slice of work.

The mission is to create a family tree/chart/artwork, going back as far as you can. This may involve some research and perhaps a trip to one of the internet sites that assist with this – there are some great free ones out there! You may then begin to compile your tree. This may be done on a computer, freehand, painted with portraits, with bright colouring pens, using photographs and interesting slices of information about each person. Work on creating something interesting to look at and to explore.

If for any reason this feels uncomfortable or you are unsure of your family background, you can take this opportunity to create a new family tree, starting with you as the head of the family, leaving plenty of space for whoever comes next (and any partners/current children).

Journal Prompts

- Who in my family line do I feel most connected to?

- Which branches of it do I know nothing about or feel disconnected from? Why is this? Is there anything that I can or want to do to change this?

- How might I create a family of choice from friends, family and partners?

- My vision for the family I am creating is…

 Affirmation: *I am creating greatness from the*
roots and branches of what has gone before.

Week 14
The Weight of Others' Opinions

There is something about pregnancy that brings people's unsolicited opinions to the fore. Those who wouldn't deign say a word about your decisions, work or choice of partner, will suddenly have strong words to say about your pregnancy, your body, how to be a parent and in particular, how they would or would not do it.

These uninvited words stem from a culture and society whose focus is usually derogatory towards those same subjects. Comments come couched in negative phrases, unhelpful responses, and projections from their lives into yours that neither align nor are healthy. These conversations, often one way, and without thought for what you need or want to hear, can feel horribly toxic.

You may have already experienced some of these types of conversations. For the most part, across all my pregnancies, people have been polite, appropriate and kind. Occasionally though you will meet with painful assaults of verbal diarrhoea that can leave you feeling attacked, or simply low about where you are at. It is important to remember that the people spouting ugly opinions or words at you are often very much reflecting their own experiences, capabilities and regrets in your direction. Whatever their experiences of these things may be, it does not mirror yours. You choose your experience, and the weight of another's opinion should not affect nor dent your confidence in it.

Another form of opinion can come in a less clear way. You may be having a loving, warm conversation with somebody trusted and kind. You are being vulnerable, they are respectful, and they say something during the back and forth that sticks in your gut. It could be an entirely neutral comment, or something that is meant well. For some reason it feels like a slap, and it replays in your mind. Even the most inane and inoffensive of words can become like hot glue poured on your heart.

As you start to share your pregnancy news more widely you may be privy to the machinations and other people's well-meant opinions on what you are doing with your life. Often these thoughts are delivered mindlessly, and you are expected to simply absorb this like a sponge. It can catch you off guard and you may find yourself compromising your stance or laughing along at your own expense to ease the situation.

These words can make you feel vulnerable and exhausted, judged and defensive. This week we will be focusing on ways to counter the weight of other people's opinions and centre our own feelings and thoughts as the prominent energy and dynamism of this pregnancy. We will discover ways to protect your heart from the words others throw your way, and to dislodge them after a barbed comment has struck. This will serve you well into parenthood, allowing you to focus on what feels right and good for you, whilst disregarding anything that does not fit, or that feels sticky, irksome or in any way alien to the life you are rightfully and mindfully choosing to create.

 # Meditation:
Heart Healing Visualisation

Take some breaths, close your eyes and make yourself comfortable.

Sit calmly for a few moments and bring yourself to your centre, to your inner experience.

Visualise a heart-shaped temple or cathedral appearing in front of you. It has many entrances, many doorways and staircases leading between each. Approach slowly and choose your stairs and door. Move towards your choice, climb the stairs, open the door and let yourself in.

As you move through the rooms, chasms and tunnels of this space, you recognise it as your own heart. You are here to cleanse and clear this space. Wander the chambers, feeling the pulsating of love, blood and emotion all around you, you may see little arrows and barbs piercing the walls. Imagine pulling them out, unhooking them and kissing any wounded areas that are left. The wounds heal up and you feel more complete, more whole and more engaged with your own knowing and understandings.

Continue to walk through the temple that is your heart. You may find it useful to repeat this mantra as you move around imagine yourself cleansing and clearing this space:

"I bring love, peace and strong self-knowing to my emotional centre."

Repeat this as often as you like or use your own words. You may like to imagine yourself conducting ritual, burning cleansing oils or herbs and singing as you move through your heart.

As you leave the space, throw the barbs and arrows to the winds, trusting they will be taken and transmuted. Your heart is released and free to experience the world as you choose to see it.

Take a few deep breaths, holding yourself in your arms with love. When you are ready open your eyes and return to the room.

 ## Soulful Practice: *Protection*

The clamour of attention around this time can be a lot. Whilst parts of it are to be delighted in, even the most wonderful of experiences may leave you drained and vulnerable to other people's moods and energies. To protect you from this we will be setting up and repeating psychic protection every single day.

This is surprisingly easy and will allow you to create etheric boundaries to keep you safe from any verbal violations or attacks. Even if such things come your way, with your protection in place, you will not feel them so harshly.

At the start of each day, before you interact with anyone, take a few moments to undertake this little ritual. This might be undertaken in the shower, imagining the water washing away any unhelpful energies, or simply sat somewhere peacefully for a minute or two.

Imagine yourself surrounded by a glowing light. You can call the light in, or imagine it descending like a bubble upon you. You may wish to repeat ... these words mentally or verbally:

"I am safe, I am protected, I attract only supportive and wholesome interactions."

Breathe deeply into this intention. Repeat as necessary.

To add layers of protection to this you may wish to burn some incense, sage or Palo Santo and walk through the smoke. There may be a song that makes you feel powerful which you play in the background. Or perhaps you could spritz yourself with protective essential oils or flower essences.

Undertake this ritual on purpose each day to set up full scale protection of your soft and vulnerable inner world.

Creative Practice:
Releasing Others' Opinions

There may be a rumble of feeling building within, a whole host of ups and downs clamour in your thoughts and feelings. The Creative Practice this week is to work these emotions and ideas into a piece of creativity. This can be whatever you like and in a medium you feel comfortable with.

If you like to write, then set about a rant or a poetic stream of consciousness. One that is not prompted by any questions, but that allows you to follow the thoughts until they are all represented onto the page. If you like to paint or draw then express yourself in this way, with colour, pen marks or pencil shading.

You may like to try something new: dance it out with loud music in the kitchen, or sing to your favourite belters at the top of your voice until your throat is scorched and something within has shifted.

Whatever creative task you choose, do it until any heavy feelings have left. Type it, walk it, plant it out of yourself and leave it where it is. Use your creative process this week to liberate your soul from any pent-up frustrations and unwelcome attentions that have come your way.

Journal Prompts

- What has been the loveliest response to your pregnancy?

- Have there been any responses that you have found tricky or challenging? Why is this?

- How did you respond in the moment? On reflection how do you wish you had responded? Allow this to play out in your imagination or write out what you wish you had said and perhaps read it aloud.

- How have other people's words affected your own wellbeing recently or in the past?

 Affirmation: *I reject and return any*
words that cause me harm.

Week 15
Challenges are Purpose

Pregnancy provokes challenge like nothing I have experienced before. There is a universe inhabiting your womb and it spirals out to affect you, your life, your family and inwards back to itself. The weight of this, and the events it causes and leads to, can feel utterly crippling at times.

Challenges, in whatever form they arise, are most difficult because of the fear that arises alongside them. It is often not the challenge itself that is the issue. That can be dealt with, action can be taken, one foot can be placed in front of the other. Rather, the fear around the possibilities our mind presents us with can surpass the challenge itself and become deeply ingrained blocks and limitations.

As you move further into this pregnancy, I would like to take the opportunity to explore the challenges that arise as part of the purpose that you are living. We all tend to see challenges as something that are unfair and righteously should not occur. Yet they do, repeatedly. If we were to review our lives objectively, we might allow an opinion to form that it is our challenges that have helped us to grow, and to become who and what we are. Still, we continue to baulk at the arrival of new challenging situations. Like young children we stick out our lower lips and declare them 'not fair'.

Perhaps the 'not fair' is exactly what is needed: it forces us down paths we didn't want to walk, yet here we learn new things. Maybe that learning is about our resilience, possibly it is about our ability to handle things, or yet still, it may be that we start to remember just who we really are as a result. Challenges, grotesque and difficult as they can be, are a part of our story, a necessary and important part. They gift us purpose and they help us to evolve. Challenges are exactly what we need, and are part of the exquisite tapestry of the moment we are in.

This week you will explore this concept more, for pregnancy can be fraught with challenges that you wish you could slide out and away from. Each bout of hardship carries with it a map, a code to your own growth and magnificence. Each challenge leads you to exactly where you need to be.

Meditation: *Tend to Your Wounds*

No matter how much I sing the anthem of challenges being purposeful, it does not negate the fact that challenge provokes and causes wounds. This may be the sparking of old pain, the anxiety of what might come, and the reality generated by painful or difficult circumstances. Whilst we may bravely declare a challenge to be a turning point, or a power moment, it is also often a cause of tears and tantrums. This is perfect, it is part of processing and growth. This week our meditation will focus on soothing the arising wound and finding ways to calm ourselves in an emotional circus.

Breathe deeply and lie comfortably. Let's go on a journey together to a place of healing and celestial offerings.

Imagine you are floating on a boat, the direction of which you have no control over, allowing it to flow wherever it takes you down a beautiful river in a jungle or through a forest. You feel safe and protected, and you recognise the journey you are on to be one of healing and closure. Perhaps you realise you have been on this boat some time, floating repeatedly into the unknown, through ups and downs, good and bad. Maybe at times you have steered, at other times the wind and waves have taken you. The momentum has slowed, and whatever you have lived through, or are living through, there is time now for regrouping, for healing, for tending to your wounds.

Imagine your boat floating towards the mouth of a cave, you lie back and allow yourself to be drawn into this sacred sanctum at the foot of a mountain, colossal in power and natural healing ability. The cave is not dark as you might expect, but lit up by millions of shining crystals, each exuding its own light and energy. The cave hums with their vibration, forming its own sound at a pitch and intensity that matches your highest potential. Every breath you take pulls in the energy of love, and of clarity. Your whole essence reverberates in unity with the cave. You start to feel whole, as if your parts are being returned. Your fractured energy, heart and mind is coming together, being reborn in ways that elicit warm feelings within. You feel held. You feel energised. You revel in clarity and knowing. Allow the energy of the cave to settle around and within you, to return all your power to you and evolve you past yourself to the next level of being.

Allow this space to be one of regaining your totality. Know that this energy will stay with you for some time even after you leave the sanctity of the cave. It will flood your veins with restorative invigoration. Where the wounds sit, emotionally, mentally and physically, you start to feel strengthened.

As the energies subside your boat floats through the cave and out the other side. You recognise that you can't go back the way you came in, the journey is forward, to new terrain. The air here feels fresh and ripe with possibility. Take several long slow breaths. Imagine your boat mooring up on a small beach. Disembark and stretch your limbs, move your body, allow restoration to greet your toes all the way to your scalp. Whenever you are ready, allow the images to drop away and come back to your space, your body and your day. Open your eyes, regroup and enjoy a nice long drink of water.

Soulful Practice:
Bringing Yourself to the Moment

When obstacles and challenges arise in life, our instinct is often to jump ship, to avoid them or to freeze up and hope they go away, all of which avoid the necessary energy of engaging with the problem. There is little to be gained from those approaches, and yet we return to them over and over, with hopes that a little aversion and avoidance will do the trick.

If we are to believe that there is purpose in our challenges, then we must believe too that we can choose to have faith in them. We can slant the situation to try to see the potential it holds, or at least the lesson. Sometimes difficulties feel so insurmountable that we can't get a grip on their purpose until many years later. At times, we may need to also recognise that there is no purpose in the horrors we experience. But, as a client of mine recently suggested, we can find one, declare one, make a purpose out of the darkest scenario, we can choose to imbue our trauma with power if we wish when we are ready.

Practice this week having faith in your challenges, for they will come no matter what. Some things will be small fry, easily manageable with a little attention and action. Other things may be bigger and harder to tackle, yet if we show up with faith that the circumstances hold something for us, we are opening routes of understanding that may just make the circumstance less frightening or stressful.

As you meet with difficulty this week, do so from the perspective that it is unavoidable and that it holds life within it. Whether you are met with a traffic jam, an unruly colleague, a financial obstacle or another complaint in a long list of dreary worries from friends and family, now is the time to hold space for it.

Allow the challenge to happen and bring your whole self to it, not in anger or frustration, but in honestly held knowing that this moment is as important as happier ones. Let the difficulty play out and do its thing: observe, react slowly and be present.

Creative Practice: *Release Frustration*

Holding space for difficulties and challenges can be consuming, taking up energy and space within our physicality. To release this, we must move physically. Because what you are holding may be outside your normal daily life, the quest is to move differently. Of course, you may be limited at present, which becomes challenging itself. The solution is to move creatively, to move purposefully, to move with the intention of disengaging your frustration.

To release pent up feelings, a run, energetic dance, hot yoga or a good kickboxing session would perhaps be something you could usually do. However, being pregnant tends to bar those, unless you have been consistently training in those arenas.

Our Creative Practice this week will be a movement you mindfully design yourself. It can be super simple, or more complex. Here are some examples:

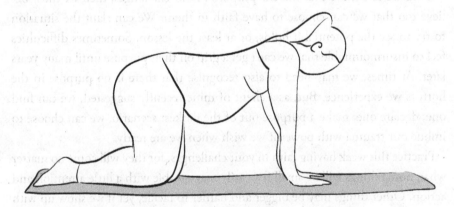

- Sit, taking deep breaths, pulling air into your body then breathing it out fiercely whilst pushing your arms away.
- Stand listening to invigorating music and sway side to side with your arms wrapped around you, pulling in love for self on the in breath and pushing out vexation on the out.

- When you wake in the morning, give your body a good jiggle and shake, imagining all the worry and concern being thrown off your body, much like water is shaken from a dog's fur.

Find your movement, repeat it every day, bring music and sound to the project. These are just ways to actively work with your body.

Journal Prompts

- What are my current challenges allowing me to experience?
- How have difficult times made me a better person?
- What would I change about this situation if I could (and would I really)?
- What one thing might I do today to be more present and engaged with the challenges I am experiencing?

 Affirmation: *I am exactly where I need to be.*

Week 16
Trusting Your Instincts

Intuition is something often associated with women, especially mothers. Instincts and intuition cover much of the similar ground – an unconscious way of knowing. But there are subtle differences too. Instinct is a term used by biologists and psychologists to refer to the innate biological knowing and behaviours displayed by any animal, such as nesting, migration or mating. Intuition is a term used for a feeling or knowing we get about whether something is safe, good or trustworthy or not, a decision usually come to not by rational, logical thought, but by gut instinct or the unconscious mind.

As humans often we forget that we are animals. Pregnancy is where our mammalian instincts come to the fore. Being pregnant both instinct and intuition kick in, in full force: our biological and spiritual instincts are doing everything they can to keep us and our babies safe. We are learning vast amounts of new behaviours and developing greater awareness without even being fully aware of it. In our culture our thinking brains are where our modern education system puts all its focus. But before these modern brains developed, we were still birthing mammals. Our instincts, especially around birth and parenting, are ancient and know nothing of fashions in birthing and childcare.

I spent time with a new mother recently, she turned to me and said, with a look of desperate resignation on her face, "Why did no one tell me how hard it is?" I felt for her and, as we got to chatting, I realised the reason it was so hard for her, was that she was desperately trying to toe the line and keep everyone happy. She was trying to follow all the advice dispensed by professionals and friends and was attempting to make it fit her baby and herself, whilst overriding her own instincts and intuition.

Within our conversation I told her that everything she was doing was right, but only if it felt that way. Nobody will give you permission to feel your own way through raising a baby. Nobody but you. And by golly is that permission important. For everyone will have an opinion, and the weight of expectation will squash your instinct if you allow it to. Working on giving yourself permission to parent and love and lead in your own unique way, right now, is deeply important.

My advice, and the only advice I will offer in this book when it comes to parenting, is this: trust your instincts and your intuition. Do what feels good and do what feels like love.

Pregnancy and motherhood are a huge exercise in self-trust and intuition. My first child was my most vital mission and quest in empowering my inner knowing. To do that, with a fragile life in my hands, felt immense. Yet it was only when I started to do things my way, to satisfy my urges, to do with my baby what my heart and gut told me to, that parenting became easier. Only when I chose to favour my instinct over and above the experiences and bookish knowledge of others, did I hit a smooth and easier stride. I fully recommend it.

I hope that the practices throughout this book will help you carve out that intuition so that you can, when the time is right, connect to your choices powerfully, and begin to release the opinions and ways of doing that do not align with you. That for me was the answer to raising a child happily and with minimum stress, blissfully even at times. This week we are working on starting to explore that intuition and make it more prominent in your everyday.

Meditation: *Animal Instincts*

Journey with me to an 'imaginary' world where you will connect with talking animals, wise old birds and trees, rocks and flowers that seem to know you.

Play some restful music, or if you have it, repetitive jungle drums would be wonderful. Move into your usual meditative space and positioning. Take three breaths and allow yourself to drop out of your everyday rhythms and into a beautiful inner space.

Look around and note the exuberance of life, you may be in a jungle or a busy woodland. Take time here to notice and watch the creatures: observe a mother bear protect her cub, a newborn deer take its first stumbling steps, courting birds building a nest, butterflies seeking out flowers with the most nectar. They trust their instincts and follow them. Just as you are learning to trust and follow your own instincts.

You are in this space to meet a nature dwelling guide that wishes to walk with you for the rest of your pregnancy. Before you conjure this being to the fore, you may wish to explore a little, noticing the life that dwells within this amazingly imaginative space. Recognising that whilst this comes from you, and is part of you, it also has aspects of the divine rolling through. Allow your mind and inventiveness to merge with what comes. You don't need to be in control of the action, allow it to play like a film and be with it, as you witness it.

Take time to be here and introduce your energy to this place, perhaps chatting to the wildlife you meet along the way. Until eventually you come to a clearing. It is here you will await your power animal. Try not to have expectations. This animal is whatever is needed and necessary currently. You may desire something magnificent and receive something humble, or vice versa. Each creature holds wisdom, give them permission to be what they are no matter their guise. As they come to you, allow them to take you on a journey through their world, to show you sights and to speak with you. Enjoy this unique interaction and spend quality time allowing this to unfold…

When the time with your animal feels ready and ripe to be over, wish them goodbye with love, and perhaps, with words of request for how they might help you moving forward. Trust that unseen, they will play a part in your personal progression. Then find your way back to your entry point and return to your everyday world.

Once you have reassimilated to your body and space, open your eyes, and use this time to make some notes. What happened? What was your animal? I recommend you run a search on your animal and come to know it in new ways. How does it live? What are its skills and talents? What does it eat? Learn about the types of families it lives in or the way it exists on planet Earth. What does it symbolise in different cultures? Take this information as reflective of things you may need to work with as you move forward in your life.

 ## Soulful Practice: *Intuition & Instinct*

Our focus in this week's Soulful Practice will be on digging for and surfacing the voice of your instinct and intuition. I encourage you to create an energy of mindfulness in all you do. Let your mind and heart wander and do their thing, but witness what it is they are doing. Are you experiencing anxious voices? If so, what sits beneath that anxiety? Is there a voice buoying you up somewhere within? Can that voice be accessed and sourced?

Often people are unsure what their intuitive voice sounds like. Here is a key that I find vital in classifying whether what I am feeling is intuition or something else:

• Intuition feels like hope, it feels like unexpected direction and heartfelt knowing. When intuition strikes it is clear, it is known, and it makes sudden sense, it can also feel deeply joyful as solution and clarity bubble as if from nowhere.

• Anything that is not intuition will feel uncertain, fearful, anxious, frightening or in need of some permission or affirmation.

Similarly, you may have become distracted and uncertain of what your instinct is. There may be some overlapping spaces between instinct and intuition, though the purest instinct sits in a very 'immediate' space. Perhaps it surfaces as a quick reaction to danger, or a suspicion of a funny smell or taste.

As a mother I have found instinct arising in some unexpected occurrences. Waking a few moments before my babe and unable to go back to sleep knowing they are about to cry out for me, which a few minutes later, they do.

I've also had the bizarre experience of being able to smell when my young children are tired. I found myself, without thinking or guidance sniffing my children's heads when they were young and sometimes finding a slight burning smell emanating. This was unconscious, but when I whiffed it, I knew they needed a nap. This happened without thought, just as you will find superhuman strength, reaction and speed occur without planning when your child wanders towards a road…

• Instinct doesn't always give you time to think, it moves through like lightning, or raises up as a fundamental understanding or animalistic 'tuning in'. It can't be practiced, but it should be trusted.

I find that some of my most profound 'meditative' understandings stemming from my intuition come in moments of gentle action. Make space for these. Such activities might include: general domestic work, driving, taking a long walk, swimming, switching off your phone and just 'being', taking a shower, gardening, whilst occupying a moment of silence to eat or rest. Take note of how your inner world shifts when your hands and body are busy, and your mind is gently occupied. This is a perfect recipe for intuition and instinct to bubble to the surface and tell you how you are really feeling.

Take this week to enter your thoughts and feelings and start to sort through the internal experiences you are having. Choose the thoughts that feel healthy, good and hopeful. Those that feel difficult can be swapped out for the more bountiful and dreamy ones. As you do this, notice how your intuitive hopeful thoughts land you in a place of certainty and confidence. Pursue these, let them become your normal, as you consciously make efforts to lay anything less than intuition to the side.

Creative Practice: *Basic Instincts*

This week we're going to be observing instincts, first in other creatures and then in ourselves:

- Take yourself to a zoo, nature park or farm, watch the birds in your park or garden, watch your pet or even watch a nature documentary. Observe the instincts that govern the behaviours of these different animals, watch how they follow them without second guessing.

- Take time to observe yourself and the instincts that you exhibit: when you flinch away from something hot or dangerous, when you jump when someone surprises you, when you feel drawn to comfort someone in distress.

- Follow one of the instincts you have experienced this week in your creative work – paint, write, move in a way that is fully driven by your instincts this week. Observe how it feels to create in such an instinctive way.

Journal Prompts

- When did I last pay close attention to my personal intuition? Write about what happened.

- What happened last time I ignored my intuition and how might this be an interesting lesson?

- What does intuition feel like for me?

 Affirmation: *I am spirit, I am intuition, I am.*

Week 17
Clarity

For the nine months of pregnancy you are mostly free from addictive behaviours, stimulants and mood-altering substances. You are on a mission, hurtling towards a date you have little or no control over, with precious cargo in tow. The combination of these factors does wonders to focusing us on what really matters. Pregnancy can be a trip towards greater clarity in your life: becoming clearly you, clear in heart and mind, clear from the expectations and efforts of others, a higher version of yourself than the more muddied person you may have been before this one thing – your pregnancy – changed everything.

Clarity comes in moments and is too suddenly affected by events, words, actions and contradictions. I'm sure you can think of times when your peace has been interrupted by news, facts, opinions and results… Clarity is a close friend of intuition, and when it dawns, it feels innate, like you always knew something (even though knowing seems an impossibility). Much like intuition, it can feel divinely gifted, as if it has been dropped upon you by some other force. The more you work upon connecting to your intuition, your inner story and feeling, the closer clarity comes.

In pregnancy some things may seem much clearer than others, and this is peppered by distracting facts and numbers, often gifted by well-meaning experts, nurses, doctors, family and friends. Clarity allows for the insight to dive and delve through all this information, and find a pearl of inner knowing, of inner truth. This pearl tells us that everything is exactly as it is meant to be, no matter how fraught or unexpected, this is the journey, and the stillness within holds some space to settle and find a path forward.

In pregnancy the future remains unknown, yet the feelings we use to guide us are often heightened. We can, given energy and moments of inner reflection, become quite 'seer' like. Some cynical folks may view this as being over-sensitive or hormonal perhaps, yet there is truth in these heightened emotions that you may not usually explore.

As you move forward in pregnancy, consider every day an opportunity to discover your truth more deeply. I write this following a call from an antenatal nurse steeped in fear, with a likelihood of more testing to gain medical 'clarity' in my pregnancy. I cried for an hour after, trying to assimilate the possibilities and obstacles that I may or may not be facing. Then I took my own medicine, I sat for a while with what I felt soulfully, bodily and internally to be true. That truth sat in hope, a vision of the future that resides within me and the possibility that all can be well. I can confirm that in time all was well, and my intuition trumped the fear-laden statistics I had been forced to contemplate.

Clarity is found on the other side of disagreements, obstructions, fatigue, pain and love. Find your clarity in self-compassion and following your heart, in the intrigues that capture you and the new things that tickle your soul. You find it when faced with difficulty and danger. Just as you may find it by the sea, in a lover's arms, or the kindness of a stranger. There is a crystal-clear truth within you that is couched in love and padded out by stillness. This is the place we seek this week.

Meditation: *Beneath the Noise*

This meditation is more akin to traditional meditation. We are not going on a visualised journey, but rather we are giving over to peacefulness. We are aiming to get beneath the 'noise' of our own minds and sink into a more passive and ease-filled state of being despite the busyness of the world outside.

This meditation may be best done before a nap or bedtime, allowing you to still the inner and outer sounds before dropping into rest. It is a practice that will come in useful for labour, where hospital rooms often have many repetitive noises which can distract you from dropping down into your centre.

Rather than listening to music, you are encouraged to have some other background sound, a fan, white noise, rain sounds or whale sounds playing to accompany you. Such sounds are accessible on free apps, YouTube, or via your usual music player. It is sensible to block at least an hour out for this meditation, as you may find that once the moment takes you over, that it is rather enjoyable, and time will fly by.

Take a moment to connect to the breath, to relax your body, and to give over to softness.

Give yourself permission to just be. As thoughts arise, observe them, and let them pass. Any distracting noises in your mind can be dealt with by returning to the breath and focusing on the repetitive sounds outside of you. You may also like to occasionally bring your attention to your body, seeking out hot spots of tension and breathing purposefully towards them, with the theme of softening over and over. Make sure you are comfortable, snuggle up in blankets and pursue slowness purposefully.

This meditation should pull you into a graceful form of rest, one in which your mind moves out of the way and allows for inner explorations. You may not remember what these inner explorations were when you come round, however you may feel assured that they felt empowering and refreshing, as if some pearls of wisdom have been deposited just outside of your grasp. Trust that whilst this magic remains unknown to your conscious mind, it will weave its way to you now that you have allowed it surface.

Rest in this as long as is necessary.

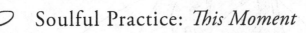

Soulful Practice: *This Moment*

Making ourselves present for clarity is extremely powerful. This means dropping thoughts of things which happened in the past, and things that may happen in the future. This can be difficult. Many of these past- and future-based thoughts have become habitual and we don't realise we are entertaining them. We walk around our lives making choices and establishing our understandings based upon the mythical, biased and wishy-washy evidence in our heads. It is hard for clarity to interrupt the strength of our feelings as they relate to past and future concerns.

Our Soulful Practice this week is to be in the moment. A favourite of many spiritualities, 'being in the moment' is a practice that can change everything. It may take years to establish a true connection to 'right here, right now', and yet, we must start somewhere.

This week we begin seeking presence and clarity. This can be done in numerous ways, and I will set out simple examples here:

The breath. The breath connects us to now. Whenever you find your mind waddling off into past or future territory, bring yourself back to three breaths. Make them long and slow. Hold your hand on your heart and determine to be with the moment: breathe into this moment. You will feel so much more focused after these three deep breaths.

Exist in your body. Being in the body is a beautiful distraction from the mind, which tends to wander: walk, move, make, do, find ways to occupy your space that is mindful and keeps your energy flowing.

Inquiry. When anxiety about the future drops in, or you find yourself perusing the past and making assumptions, ask yourself, "how much of this is based on my current reality?" Interrupt your thoughts and drop into what is happening now.

You may also want to ask yourself, "how do I feel right now?", then examine your response. Is it based on things that once happened or of hope/fear for what may happen? Find the parts that are relevant for today. Be with them, let them infuse the situation with truth.

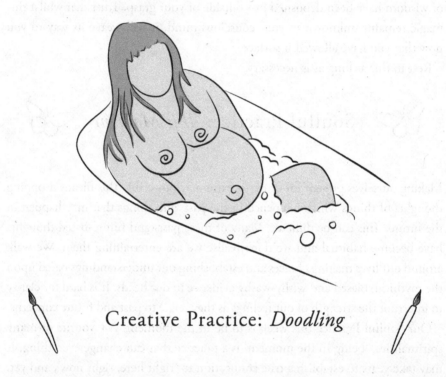

Creative Practice: *Doodling*

One thing that is sure to clear my mind and bring me to the moment is a spot of doodling. I have, throughout my life, found it to be the most wonderful distraction from all kinds of rigours. My schoolbooks were works of art, full of line drawings, waves, eyes and simplistic pages filled with dots and crosses.

To this day, I find that doodling focuses me. Whenever I am on a call with a client, their notes will be decorated with flowers, wiggly worms in top hats with multiple legs and smiley faces. To the outside world it may look like I was not fully present, but the act of flowing with ink to paper, whilst listening and responding, is deeply calming.

This week I ask you to create the circumstances in which you would like to doodle, and to give yourself permission to do this. I remember in my youth, when all we had for a telephone was a landline, my mum's address book was filled with my scribblings (she made me buy her a new one it became so graffitied!). When in life have you felt the urge to doodle? Perhaps phone someone for a long conversation but do it with a pen and paper to hand. Instead of scrolling your phone whilst watching the TV, you might swap the device for a blank sheet of paper and a beautifully flowing ink pen.

Part of the magic of doodling is often that it isn't the main thing you are doing, it's a side effect of something else. There is no desired outcome or purpose to it. Doodling is creativity for the sake of it. It connects to the primal within and takes to the page almost by surprise, transforming thoughts into images in fun and beautifully unimportant ways.

 ## Journal Prompts

- When I sit in stillness with no distraction, I start to feel the following things...

- How do I actively repress these feelings?

- What habits do I indulge to zone out from my feelings?

- What are these feelings trying to tell me?

- How might I honour and make space to feel and witness my inner world moving forwards?

 Affirmation: *I know precisely who I am.*

Week 18
Dream Life

In pregnancy you may find that your sleep is either deeply disturbed – with early hours trips to the toilet or a baby looking to party whilst you're trying to sleep, or deeply interesting, full of psychedelic dreams…or perhaps both of those things on a loop!

I have found that within this pregnancy my sleep life has been replete with vivid dreams, the type that feel like a movie is playing out and I get to be both star and a witness within it. The feelings provoked are intense and outside of my daily experience, and yet, there are reflections of myself – my innermost hopes and fears – cropping up in every interaction and aspect of the dream. If I compare the plotlines of my dreams to the events of my daily life, I can see echoes and reflections of the conflicts and contradictions arising, the hopes and the reality, the daily normality colliding and clashing with this cinemascope of imagination. There is truth sitting like a kernel within each crazy dream episode.

Dreams also have the potential to bring forth a more direct connection to spirit. My mother-in-law has visited my dreams often in this pregnancy. She is still with us in life, though tragically her mind is trapped in a terrible state of late dementia. Just a few years ago she was so capable and very much in love with my children. Lately she crops up in dreams in good health and so happy to see me – evidence to me that she is on some level aware of what is happening and finding ways to bring herself to a pregnancy that she would've been so excited about. Just as occasionally my grandfathers or grandmother will appear unexpectedly, bringing love and connection, as if they had never passed. Dreams are a space where a clear connection to the spiritual world and the love of people we have known can easily infiltrate.

Whilst dreams can be had at any stage of life, these pregnancy dreams seem much more loaded than usual and tend to have a much bigger impact on us in our waking lives, often remembered for years to come. At a time when we may be becoming more physically limited in our daily lives, there is freedom and surprise in really allowing ourselves to be fully engaged in our dream worlds. I recommend it fully!

This week you are invited to explore the depths of your dreams purposefully and with a view to expanding and evolving your awareness of self...

Meditation: *Dream Meditation*

This week your meditation practice will focus on returning consciously to your dreams. Working alongside the soulful and creative aspects offered this week, you will take time to ponder the aspects of your dreamlife.

This may be done by sitting consciously with flowing music and deep breaths and allowing your mind to wander to elements of your dream, seeing what comes up, or where they may go...

You might also like to take your memories of a dream and walk with them. Often walking allows us to shut down the critical parts of our brain and look at problems or situations differently. Take your dream memories for a walk and see if you remember more, or if the dreams expand somehow, gifting you deeper self-awareness.

If you wake early and have time where you don't have to get up, then try to go back to sleep and return to the dream. This is such a beautiful indulgence, and even if you don't revisit the dream, you may well start a new one!

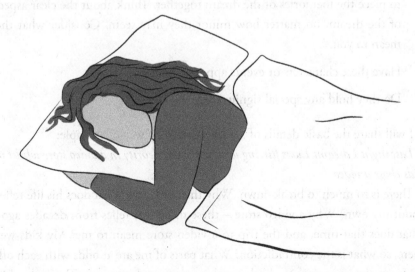

Soulful Practice: *Dream Diary*

Keep a dream diary and record your dreams. Dreams are a portal into our unconscious. The stories and events that play out through them tend to tell us a great deal about ourselves. Making efforts to understand your own dreams can help new dreams come along, with more vivid and clear personal understandings. Even if your dreams are whispery and hard to remember, taking a few minutes to try to recall small details each day is a step towards greater detail coming to fruition on future nights.

It can be easy to ignore your dream life and write it off as the imagination let loose in sleep. Yet, you may find that even with a little amateur sleuthing, your dreams make some kind of sense. They reflect something about yourself that you can explore or accept. This can be helpful, or, at the least, interesting.

Start your dream diary this week by going to sleep with a pen and journal by your bed. If you wake at any time in the night or morning with a dream fresh in your mind, write it all down. Not only the main story, but the smaller details...

- Where were you?

- How did you feel?

- What items/people/places/things were involved?

- After the dream is written down as much as possible, take a moment to start to piece the memories of the dream together. Think about the clear aspects of the dream, no matter how minor they may seem. Consider what they mean to you.

- Have these characters or events appeared before?

- Do they hold any special significance to you?

I will share the basic details of a recent dream by way of example:

Last night I dreamt I was flirting with a minor celebrity in a video store whilst my kids chose a video.

There is so much to break down. Why this celebrity? What does his life reflect about my own? Why a video store – these things are relics from decades ago – what does that time, and the trip to a video store mean to me? My kids were there, so what is the contradiction? What parts of me are at odds with each other? It may be important to check out themes across dreams too. This is the third night in a row I have dreamt about flirting with a different random celebrity, each time in different circumstances that otherwise I should perhaps have been giving my attention to… Are your dreams repeating in theme, feel or energy?

Though a good book on dreams may be helpful, I'd encourage you to work on your dreams by sourcing your own understandings first. Play and come up with your own theories. At a time when physically you may be feeling limited, this new spectrum of dream adventure is a gorgeous soulful insight into who you are becoming…

Creative Practice:
Capture Your Dreams

Dreams can feel like something that happen to us. I believe that by working with them, we might start to go deeper, perhaps experience some choice and freedom within our dreams and begin to interact with our own growth and healing through them.

Your Creative Practice this week is to try to take creative control of your dreams. Following the work set out in the Soulful Practice section is the first step. But other ways are suggested here…

- Upon going to bed, ask your dreams for an answer or an adventure. Go to bed expecting something intriguing to happen. Try this every night for the week and see where it takes you!

- Base your creative practices around your dreams. Draw, sing, paint, dance, write or grow something based around some theme of your dream. Bring what occurred in your head into reality in some way.

- Sleep with a crystal under your pillow: moonstone, amethyst and a simple clear quartz may help provoke connective, interesting dreams, whilst also offering protection and soothing properties.

- Dab some essential oils on your wrist: lavender is famously known for prompting good sleep, whilst frankincense and rosemary may help you find spiritual connection and clarity within your dream life.

- Pull an oracle or tarot card as a guide to your dream: pull the card just before going to sleep, then invite the energy in whilst also asking your guides/angels/higher self for protection.

- Speak to trusted friends about your dreams and get their take on the elements you remember. You don't have to agree, but it may be fun to explore their opinions.

Dreams are a space of great creativity waiting to be unearthed. By starting this daily practice of honouring and exploring them, it is likely that intriguing avenues will open in your psyche. Let this be a gift to yourself and your burgeoning family.

Journal Prompts

- Themes/characters/symbols/places that are appearing frequently in my dreams at present include...

- I remember these from...

- How do you dream – vividly, or more subtle smatterings of memories? Do you dream in colour or black and white? Do you hear voices, or music or are they silent?

- Have you had any dreams that especially stand out over your whole lifetime, from childhood and beyond? Dissect them a little here, see if in retrospect they may speak volumes to those times and situations...

 Affirmation: *My dreams entrust me with pearls of my own truth.*

Week 19
Self-Acceptance

We live in a culture that monitors what we consume and has an opinion on every aspect of our bodily changes. Pregnancy is a time of natural physical change, it can feel glorious and welcome, but at other times, physically draining and challenging. It can trigger wounds that we thought we had left behind around how we look, our age, our presentation or our weight. This pregnant change, no matter how longed for, can be tricky to navigate.

This week we will explore how the expansion of the womb, the belly and the physical body is a powerful calling to self-acceptance. There is no battle here. Though it may feel at times that there is. A battle between your appetite and your exhaustion, your previous physical ability and your current limitations. A battle between dress sizes and your intellect, a battle of self-love and self-loathing. All of this plays out alongside a desire to be happy and healthy, to provide for your growing child and to attain the mythic proportions and demeanour of a pregnant goddess.

Pregnancy can feel all-consuming, and every itch, pain and inch of growth can become an obsession. This, however, is not an opportunity to give over to societal mores about losing the baby weight, or not losing yourself. Rather I would argue it is essential in pregnancy to lose many parts of yourself so that you can come back more whole. The parts you may wish to lose may look like self-criticism, cultural expectations, the opinions of others and the belief that your body defines you as a person.

I have recently received a slew of comments from other women upon finding out I am pregnant, mostly declaring I am crazy! It is a throwaway comment that is often followed up by them commenting how they couldn't have another child, or certainly not at this age… This jump from, "Congratulations!", which I received in my thirties, to the more loaded, "Crazy!", has been deeply triggering for me. What has been activated is my own inner critic that perhaps agrees with them a little. It is crazy, I am different, this is unique, how dare I go outside of what is socially normal?

The work I am doing to counter this is recognising and redefining what "crazy" means to me, recognising that streak of "crazy" which runs through all I do and that has, in many ways, brought me a tonne of success, relentless creativity and interesting situations. I am gently holding myself through this onslaught of opinions and recognising the dire need it is provoking to accept myself and my life choices.

You may have completely different areas that become heightened when others project onto you. For me, these inner and outer judgements centred around my age. For you it might be your weight, health, career, relationship status or living situation that people judge. This week is an opportunity to hold these to the light and accept all that you are, to honour your choices and to trust that the changes you are experiencing right now, internal and external, are part of the current purpose. This purpose being something divine, honoured and held precious – even if only by our own hearts.

 ## Meditation: *Shedding Skin*

For this week's meditation I'd like you to sit in peace for five to ten minutes and consider how parts of your life are dropping away. This includes your own previously held opinions about yourself. Be with what comes up. This space is intentional and may be provoking.

Imagine you have an extraneous layer of skin, one that provides comfort, but that also weighs you down. As you consider and contemplate this protective layer, consider how it prevents you from being entirely true to yourself. It is a mask, a falsehood.

The skin that you wear is recognisable to others, and they project upon it their expectations of you. What sits beneath it is your dazzling truth, perhaps rawer and more uncertain. Visualise this old extra skin starting to drop away. Trust that the new skin underneath, albeit fresh and unworn, has layers of new understandings. Whilst part of you may wish to hold true to the familiar, there is something magical about this letting go. You are not the same as you were, the change is unnerving, but you must accept this new layer, this new depth, this new version of you.

Continue to imagine allowing your protective hard old skin to drop away. Focus on the dazzling light of your fresh new baby skin. How soft and vulnerable it is. Recognise that the protection you need is not found in hardening, but in accepting yourself in all your vulnerable choices, decisions and quirks. Hold yourself tight and offer yourself acceptance and love.

Sit with this releasing of the old for as long as it feels potent. When you are ready, feel yourself held in your new skin, breathe deeply to reinvigorate your day, and return to your moment.

Soulful Practice:
Why You Are Wonderful

This week our Soulful Practice focuses on dropping all negativity, and bringing your attention to things you can see and understand about yourself to be wonderful. Not things that are 'okay' or 'good enough' but reasons why you are spectacular.

Begin a list. Head this list in your journal with 'Why I Am Wonderful'.

Start wherever you can. Present your own compelling list of magic about yourself including: things you have done; achievements; amazing experiences you have enjoyed; moments of laughter; friendships; family; your heartfelt and strong opinions; physical aspects of yourself that you admire; behaviours and patterns you are proud of; challenges you have overcome... Let this list be fully exhaustive and return to it often throughout the week to add more and breathe into this growing representation of your own amazingness. Concentrate too on those areas that others critique, such as your loudness, your craziness or that parts of you that are quirky and different. Allow yourself to see these things as strengths.

Ask beloved family and friends for their favourite things about you (and perhaps share your favourite things about them in return). Create a love list and dedicate it to yourself.

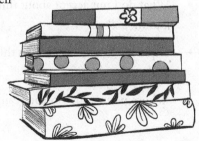

Creative Practice:
An Updated Self-Portrait

This week's practice is to create a new self-portrait of yourself as you are right now. We have undertaken this task before, though much has changed since then. In a few weeks, you have started shifting the balance of who you are, and this portrait is an exploration of that change and growth. This Creative Practice allows us to consciously hold the changes that are occurring on all levels of yourself. Whilst the task may seem repetitive, the outcome will not be. You are not the same as you were, just as in another few weeks, the changes will continue to show themselves. Let this be visible and held through your reflective self-creations.

Sit with this a few moments before putting tools to paper. This self-portrait may be a hand-drawn or painted image, a photograph or a written reflection formed in poetry or prose that captures this moment. Allow yourself to be literal or metaphorical in how you undertake this task. Bring your parts to the surface and create a mirror of what you see to be true about you at this precise time. Compare it to your previous self-portrait (if you made one) see how they differ.

Journal Prompts

- How have I changed in this pregnancy so far?

- How do I feel about my changing body?

- What do I not accept about things people have said to me? (Feel free to rant and moan!)

- Explain why your choices in this pregnancy (and life) are exactly perfect and as they should be.

- Whose permission do you really need to be yourself?

 Affirmation: *Accepting myself changes everything for the better.*

Week 20
Grandmother Wisdom

My grandmother's energy and love has been ever-present throughout my pregnancies. Even though she died a few days before I took this most recent pregnancy test, she has shown up in dreams, feelings, visions and photographs of herself popping out of stacks of paper at timely moments. I certainly feel her influence and hand in these circumstances. This is made more lovely by the fact that for at least the last ten years she was lost to a gentle dementia. Always smiling and nodding and in some kind of awareness, but not fully my grandma. Upon her death she is catching up, making herself known, being with me where she can.

It was at her home years previously that I experienced my first child embed in my womb. I pulled a tarot card and received an image of a woman holding an egg, with a baby inside it.

My American grandmother, still alive and kicking, despite a stroke, bouts of respiratory failure, ongoing heart failure, pneumonia, and general old age, and yet fully in her mind, has offered congratulations and remembers the smallest details about myself and my brother's babyhoods. Despite her physical failings and the ongoing rigours of old age, she holds so much of us within her memory and heart. This maternal line of knowing and this remembrance is a gift you are now participating in. Whilst we are the newbies, the younger of generations to undertake the task, our part in it is vital.

This week we will work with forging a creative connection with our beloved ancestors. These may be remembered loved ones, those still with us, the ancestral children that come next into the future, alongside those that we do not know, who in this moment we choose to claim.

We are all our many grandmothers, versions of her sit in our skin, as we play out some of her hopes and dreams. Similarly, our DNA, our hearts and hopes, may show up in generations going forward, carrying our essence into the future, improving upon those things we struggled with or reaching for the ambition or acclaim that we dare not.

If you have a difficult relationship with your grandmothers, or did not know them, you may choose to look back further. Call on ancient unknown people from before more recent times: those who exist in your line who are loving and good and who echo through your veins. Trust that somewhere, once upon a time, there was a soul like you, with heartfelt love in your lineage. Call on that energy, that hope and potential to infuse you. Or indeed, borrow an ancestor, there is no harm in calling forth the generic energy of a historical character, or the grandparent of a friend, or indeed any older person you admire to act as stand in.

Ancestry, known or otherwise, is the connection of self to previous (and ancient) versions of self. As we sit in a space of creating the next generation, we can call upon this moment to forge a connection more deeply, to enable power from the past, and imbue hope for the future.

Meditation:
Sitting with the Grandmothers

This is an active meditation, one in which we invite in the energies of all grandparent figures (recent or ancient) who have love and guidance for us. You may wish to undertake it with others, such as friends or a partner, or a loving relative who is open to it.

Schedule some time to simply be with this meditation. Gather any remnants of the past you may have. This could be old photographs, heirlooms, names written on paper, or if none of that is available, simply light a candle and some incense. Play gentle easy music that reminds you of the echoing past and prepare a warm drink.

Your intention is not to raise the dead – this is not a séance of any kind! Rather it is an opportunity to welcome in loving wisdom, guidance and support. This will arise in the form of insight, magical happenings and surprise guidance (and your own thoughts and dreams).

The ritualistic details of what you do within this circle is for you to decide. You may wish to drink

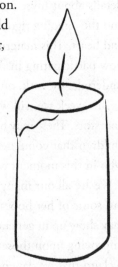

hot tea and offer up flowers. If you are feeling more active, you could write and read a list of questions and queries on your life, whilst at the same time, sending love backwards through the ages. A prayer dedicated to loved lost ones might feel powerful. You may also wish to find a song or a poem to perform in their honour.

You may open the circle of ancestral connection by stating the following:

"I welcome all loving and guiding ancestors to sit with me today, I honour you and ask for your wisdom and protection."

You may then spend some time in close eyed silence, song, poetry or even in conversation. At the end you can close the small ceremony by stating:

"Thank you for being with me, I ask for your love and guidance moving onwards, I honour your highest hopes and energies in all I do."

Bring all your focus to this meeting with the spirits of your ancestors and trust their love will find ways to filter into your everyday life.

 ## Soulful Practice: *Remembrance*

Modern-day western practices have us moving on quickly after loved ones have departed. Ancient ways would ask us to keep the energy and momentum of our beloved ones fresh. In remembrance we conjure the very best of what has gone before, we connect to the guidance of our familial line, alongside the wisdom that is carried in our DNA.

Find ways to bring a little nod to your ancestors into your everyday. This may be the tending to things that they used to grow in your garden. Last year I inadvertently grew pumpkins after my daughter's Halloween pumpkin seeded itself in a small space (where I left it out for the squirrels) – I dedicated this surprise patch to my living American grandmother.

You may wish to dedicate fresh flowers (especially ones that they used to grow or love, or that grow in profusion where they came from) or the burning of incense or oils as a daily practice to the best of your folk line. When you wake or fall asleep you may simply wish to send a greeting from your heart to the best of what was and what is to come.

Creative Practice:
Celebrating Grandmothers

This week we will be celebrating our grandmothers (and the archetype of what a grandmother is) with our creativity. If your grandmother was known for certain skills – baking, needlework, knitting, gardening, snappy dressing – do something in her honour this week. Dig out treasured items: a piece of jewellery, a letter, a photograph, a recipe book, patchwork quilt or painting. Create something inspired by it – cook a recipe from the book for your family, make a frame for the photograph...or recreate it in pencil or oil paints, make a companion quilt or repurpose the jewellery.

If you have no direct, healthy or clear connection to what your grandmother might have created or how she may have expressed herself, then lean into the energy of her generation. Explore how she or other loving women of that time might have lived, and the creative pursuits available to them. Find ways to emulate their works within your own, stitching and pasting a celebration of the past that resides within you, into your modern life.

Journal Prompts

- What are your best memories of your grandparents (or other elder figures in your life) – if you have none, what stories have been told and passed down?

- What personality traits and energies have you inherited from them?

- What have you healed in your relationships with family that will no longer affect future generations? What is left to heal?

- Do you have a vision for who beyond your immediate family you would like to act in the role of elder for your child?

 Affirmation: *I create a trail of power, healing and self-knowing for all future generations.*

Week 21
Find Your Soul Song and Sing It

Most of us have been taught to find our meaning and sense of self in our paid work regardless of how meaningful it is to us. To the outside world we are, in large part, defined by what we do, the status of our work, and how much we earn. Motherhood – an unpaid role – is little valued in our culture. Mainstream media is keen to tout the storyline that motherhood is a place where many women lose themselves. That in the milky mash-up of difficulty that it represents, we somehow give ourselves up in favour of a lesser version of self. Then, some way down the line, we 'get our bodies back', remember who we are, find the right lippy, and get back out there to our pre-children working lives.

This is, of course, a nonsense, one that purports to suggest that a role as important as raising children is destructive to the person doing the work. Let me be frank: parenthood and motherhood will disassemble you in many ways. But this is no bad thing. There are many parts of you that perhaps require change and transformation. Not one of us humans live a life unchanged. Whilst those changes can feel troubling and challenging, they are also a journey to pearlescent truth, to resilience, and to new perspectives on who you are and what you are capable of.

Pregnancy is an intensive nine-month passageway of shapeshifting, an initiation that takes you closer to your heart and bones, that finds you knocking on your own flesh and finding new doors into depths and versions of you that you hadn't realised were present. Right now, those doors are starting to crack open. What happens from here is only as difficult as your resistance. Should you choose to see this pathway as momentum towards 'new', towards 'different' and maybe even part of your purpose and soul song, then all those changes will come more easily.

Last night, on a full moon, I went to sleep with a question on my mind: "Who am I and what is my soul's purpose?" I awoke in the night with the answer: "Find your soul song and sing it." I managed to keep those words with me till morning and in reviewing them I feel they are an answer for us all. It's the advice the careers counsellor at school forgot to mention. We are all so busy trying to fit into and acclimatise to societal 'roles', that we might forget about our soul song, or neglect to think about it entirely.

As you sit with this response, at this stage of pregnancy, you might begin to feel a pull towards something, some truth you forgot, or covered up in suits, jobs, reputations and other masks. You may have even taken that 'soul song' and adapted it to fit in. The artist may have accepted a lesser version of herself, and spends hours in her office job daydreaming and doodling. The writer could have taken up advertising copywriting or found herself waist deep in dry report-writing for a governmental body. The landscape gardener may settle for a floral blouse and a nice vase of cut flowers when she has the time and extra money. The scientist or doctor may be an armchair critic of those things she finds fascinating without the gumption to commit to the training or pathway that calls.

The real loss of self is not in pregnancy or having a child, for me this is the return to self. The real loss is most often created in becoming a functional member of society and fitting in to the expectations that come with paying the bills and keeping up with the neighbours.

There is nothing worth doing except 'soul singing'. Now is the time to revisit that. Throughout the weeks of pregnancy, starting here, you will be encouraged to get back to you. To find yourself. To find yourself, particularly, within the clustered, confusing and beautiful time that is pregnancy. This book is your compass and sightline to clarity. Your life is simply a remembrance, a dedication to self and an empowerment of this physically creative stage of your life, turning some of that life force towards you, as is your right and your pleasure.

 ## Meditation: *Finding Your Soul Song*

Taking a beautiful long breath, sit with your hands over your womb, recognising this moment as an opportunity to tune into a new frequency, a place of harmony with your name on it.

You may have an awareness of the things you desire to do in life, they may also be very much on the back burner or awaiting courage. No matter where you stand in the realms of personal understanding, this meditation will help you to listen to the voice within and start to recognise that your beliefs, desires and aspirations are real, warranted and given to you so that you might do something with them.

As you give over to the breath, take this moment to dwell upon your highest wishes for life, consider the one thing you would truly like to do with your time, be this a hobby, a way of life or a working reality. Bring yourself to what it would feel like if this were true right now. Feel into the melody of life as if this were your current experience. Take time to flow into the daily grind of that wish being a reality. Who is with you, what are you doing, what is being said, what music is playing, how do you feel, and how do you flow, move, and speak?

Give yourself to this. Conjure the depths of your soul song to your heart and mind. This is a powerful act of self-recognition and of catapulting aspects of your being into possibility. This is also a way of working profoundly with manifestation, by admitting your desires and then visualising them in certainty and clarity. Diving deep into feeling them, you start to sow internal seeds of growth and magic.

Sit with the energy of your soul song, and revisit this whenever your dreams need bolstering. Each time you can imagine new aspects, new storylines and possibilities, allowing the soul song to grow alongside you.

Soulful Practice: *Ask the Question*

I asked the question and the answer I received was beautiful: "Find your soul song and sing it." This is widely applicable and profoundly true for all humans. As you sit within this steep point of change in your life, egg and sperm having done their work, having met and collided to create life, it is a beautiful time to turn a little attention back inwards, for sometimes that collision becomes all-consuming. So, whittle out a few moments for you. Take a breath in a darkened room, or out in nature, and connect to the depths of yourself. If you have faith then maybe address this question to your gods, goddesses, guides and angels, if not, then catapult this question towards your own unconscious, the inner you who 'knows'.

"Who am I and what is my soul purpose?"

Then take that question to bed with you. Place a paper and pen next to your sleeping area so that if you are awoken with insight, you can jot it down quickly. Don't worry if it doesn't come immediately. It may come in other ways. Perhaps an interesting conversation with a friend or stranger will shed light on the answer, or a sign or uncanny happening. Be on the lookout and feel into your depths. The answer may simply bubble up one day when you are distracted, a word or two that will remind you of who you are. Then grasp that, take it with you into the months ahead. Allow it to ruminate and grow and become the most important truth of you.

Creative Practice:
Photograph Your Truth

Take a photo of yourself as you are now. You are on the cusp and precipice of all kinds of change. Record this moment with a beautiful 'selfie'. Not a bump or belly shot, although do please capture your whole frame if you wish. Consciously take a photo with the knowing that this photo represents the magical between space. The version of you who existed before this pregnancy as she meets with your pregnant self. Capture your depths and your totality.

You may wish to put effort to really find yourself within this portrayal. You are welcome to involve a partner or friend to help pose, style and photograph you. This is a liminal space, and you will be glad of this image. It will act to reconnect you to parts of you that you wish to keep hold of, whilst equally starting to introduce you to some seedling of change and transition that this moment represents.

Journal Prompts

- What is my soul song? Think about what springs to mind – this may take you back to childhood and hobbies you indulged.

- What parts of my soul song have I given up and why?

- What have I been longing to explore more for myself? How might I begin to do so, even now?

 Affirmation: *I am living my soul song.*

Week 22
Rage and Anger

Pregnancy is a time of intense feelings: love, joy, excitement, grief and anger. There are few times in life when rage or anger are viewed as appropriate, especially if you happen to be female. Such feelings are culturally stuffed down to make space for more palatable emotions such as, being 'a bit miffed', or 'ever so slightly vexed'. Chances are you have felt rage and tried to think it away, to justify it entirely out of context or to simply pretend it isn't there, whilst smiling nicely and parroting, "I'm fine thanks for asking". We excuse it away (tired, hungry, premenstrual) and in doing so we rarely allow ourselves to feel it.

During this pregnancy I have found anger visiting me repeatedly. At first, I found this uncomfortable and excused myself, citing hormones and tiredness. But the more it occurred, the more frequently it sprang to my inner attention, the more I began to realise that my anger, my rage was warranted. My circumstances made anger appropriate. It was healthy anger, not out of control. It did not make me destructive. I did not become violent or aggressive (those being some symptom of toxic and unprocessed anger).

In sitting and being with my anger I recognised that it was a place of pure clarity. It didn't feel muddled or in the least confused. My anger felt appropriate, and it stemmed from being hurt and let down by a variety of different situations. I felt anger and rage, not because I was having a mental breakdown, but because I had certainty. That certainty took different forms. I was certain that I deserved better. I was certain that I am better than the behaviours, words and rejections I was witnessing. My anger elevated me above situations that otherwise I may have lost myself within.

Anger and rage, when sat with and lived with, become something quite different than the cultural expectations of them. They are strong intuitions, messages sent from a place of sincere self-love. My anger told me that I had been wronged, the situation was wrong, the treatment was wrong. My anger was a touchpaper to passion in my soul that allowed me to prioritise myself above all others.

Anger, I found, was a beautiful and helpful emotion, one that screamed, "I love myself, I am so much more than this."

In turn my responses weren't blustered and uncontrolled. By processing my anger and being with it, I found my responses became saner, they centred my well-being, and they supported my health and personal growth. The magic unknown here is that nobody has ever taught me this. It simply occurred and I came to see anger and rage as important aspects of my intuition and internal messaging. As we move through the extremes of pregnancy, anger is one extreme that has a great deal of information embedded within it. This week we explore the secret language your anger holds and begin to decipher what messages it brings.

 ## Meditation: *Sit with Your Anger*

Anger is a great motivator: it will have your home gleaming and your muscles taut as you channel it via distraction exercises into anything other than feeling it.

This week's meditation is simple. Sit in silence, for ten or fifteen minutes. Have a pen and paper to the side. Commit to focusing on your anger. Give your anger this clear and uninterrupted space to spew and vent its way to the surface. Sit with it whilst it changes form, whilst its voices rise and lower, as the tears flow or the feeling subsides. Give this time to your anger. Give it as a gift. For once let it be seen, heard and felt.

Afterwards write down, draw or express any insights. Then take yourself on a releasing walk around the block or to a local park or beauty spot. Imagine that the anger, now fully fledged and felt, drops from you with every step. Breathe deeply and admire the life and light around you in whatever way it appears. Treat yourself to a cake and warm cup of something.

At the conclusion of having meditated upon and experienced your anger, what are you left with? What message has this feeling provided for you?

 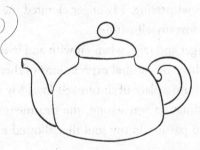

Soulful Practice: *Press Pause*

Expressing our anger as soon as it arrives is a sure-fire way to create painful and dramatic circumstances. Sitting and being patient can be enlightening. The initial response to the feeling of anger is to lash out, verbally or possibly physically. We may find ourselves screaming unkind obscenities or throwing items around or maybe we subvert our anger into passive aggression. We act quickly and believe that if only we say the thing, or act a certain way, the rage may subside, but usually it leads to more rage-inducing occurrences.

As feelings of anger arise within you this week or at other times, take pause. Once you have moved past the initial onslaught of feeling that it brings, you are left with a very different experience. You will be left with knowing, clarity and inner connection. When you stop to listen to the message that anger offers, the circumstances change.

Of course, there are circumstances in which a vitriolic and fast response is necessary, such as being attacked physically, or in any other dangerous situation. However, where your rage is induced by words, actions, unfairness or attitude, you might be surprised how a slow reaction allows for insight, wisdom and awareness of a bigger picture.

Take this week to pause and witness your fury and see what comes when the wave of vitriol has passed.

Creative Practice: *Evoking Rage*

Creativity is a great source of enlightening self-expression. It is likely that you have expressed your love, your heart, your style and your passions through your creations. Have you ever sourced and evoked rage, anger and fury into your creative work? It is a wonder and a curiosity how this might arise. As we experience our frustrations this week, we might find great solace in bringing those same tumultuous feelings to our creative path.

This week our practice is to bring the rage to the page, to sing, dance, draw or write it out of us. I simply ask that you explore the internal expression of rage as it bubbles within you and let it unfurl a new path through your work. Hold your anger as if it were a tool, choose not to launch it upon others, but first bring it to your creativity. Allow it to become real and evidential as a part of your soul-seeking words, sound and play.

You may find that your creativity under the influence of rage looks and feels different. It may choose a new format, or demand to be fed with unexpected inspiration, even a different variety of food. You may discover a softness or a yearning beneath the anger that allows you to pivot into new understandings of what really vexed you. Let this all come alive through scribbles, letters, movement, or powerfully birthed artworks and chapters.

Journal Prompts

- What message does my anger bring to me at this moment?
- What techniques do I instigate to avoid feeling my anger (and how might I become more aware of this)?
- When I think about myself being angry, I feel...
- When I give myself permission to feel and be angry, the following happens...

 Affirmation: *My anger is a vibrant messenger of my truth.*

Week 23
Rest and Balance

There comes a time in pregnancy when we recognise that our bodies are not the same as they were some months ago. For each of us this may be highlighted differently. It may be that our stamina takes a hit, or we suffer aches and pains in strange places, we may experience emotional and mental tiredness or some other unexpected and thankfully temporary phenomena.

I hit one of these walls just this week. Having felt vibrant and full of energy, I took on a mission of travel to attend my grandma's memorial, three hours away from home, with two kids in tow. I'm glad I did it, it was beautiful. The ramifications however, were not. I found myself physically floored for several days after. I had to recognise that I am not what I was only a short time ago, and that for me to remain vibrant and energetic, I must take a very different approach to my life.

Indeed, what looked like 'balance' five months ago, has now shifted to something almost unrecognisable. It is my responsibility to myself, baby and the parenting of my dependent children that I figure out what my new balance is, and how to honour it day in and day out. From this new place of shifted centres, I can grasp and properly use my remaining energy.

This week our focus is on how to adapt to the needs of our changing bodies and the changing requirements upon us to rest, work, care for others and our selves.

 ## Meditation: *Melt*

This is a beautiful easy meditation to undertake just before bed, allowing you to give over to ease and rest. This week's meditation is designed to release energy, to allow for floppy ease and marshmallow-like responses! It's a meditation I use with my children at bedtime. I call down the marshmallows (from their home in the sky) and pretend to be placing them in the bodies of my children. We do this at night-time to help them turn their bodies to a lazy mush, to let go of pent-up tension of the day and imagine their muscles giving over to luscious softness.

You can undertake this anytime, anywhere, with or without marshmallow accompaniment! I simply recommend that you find a few moments, take three large deep breaths, and then imagine all the energy that is unnecessary draining from your body, replacing the tension with velvety, cushioned, divine restfulness. Allow yourself to flop and fold in on yourself, to become mushy and soft.

Let this experience of softness simply be what it is. If you notice areas of tension, breathe the marshmallows (or feathers or softness) into your areas of firmness. Imagine them slacking and relenting. Sit with this for as many moments as you desire.

 ## Soulful Practice: *Move Slow*

This week our Soulful Practice is to purposefully deny ourselves the fast lane, and to undertake life at a snail's pace. This shift in speed is an interesting one. It may feel unnatural at first, but as the body acclimatises it recognises the opportunity to find a new rhythm and latches onto it. Whilst speed and power are the calling cards of the culture we live in, the inner culture, the divine aspect of inner truth, may well appreciate the lull in hyperactivity.

As you walk, swim, move, dance, undertake errands and live your life at reduced speed, so your thoughts and nervous system will follow pace. You give over to a different flow, one that is not fuelled by need or stress, but by trust and sloth-like tempo. All you need to do, and feel, and be will still occur.

You may like to indulge one of the following this week to help soothe and calm any fractious speed down to something a little stiller...

- Try a pregnancy yoga or yin yoga class.

- Or how about tai chi or other gentle movement class

- Join the elder women at the local gym's water aerobics or calisthenics class.

- Undertake a gentle walking meditation.

- Swim gently without a need to undertake any number of laps or speed.

- Undertake any domestic chores and errands in slow mo. Take time to be in the act of folding, sweeping, walking to the postbox or polishing. Deny the rush and let the inane boring stuff of life be lived like a soft murmur of movements and introspection.

Observe how the new slowness helps you to bubble up and brew your thoughts and plans differently.

Creative Practice:
Soulful Food

Your mission this week, in all the slowness and softness and reclaiming of balance, is to really listen to the voice within. Food can be a ritual and celebration, but at times becomes a chore or a bad habit. This week, as we reclaim the new balance, we open our minds to how this can be reflected in our food and eating. Whilst we are all guilty of grabbing the easiest, sugary snack to fuel our day, this week we look and listen internally for alternatives.

You may feel creatively compelled to a different place to shop, or to an aisle you don't usually visit. There may be a call for wetness or crunch within. As you sit to bigger meals you may wish to cook yourself something unusual or challenging from scratch or allow another to creatively cook for you.

Approach each meal this week as if it were an artwork of possibility. Each item you consume will fuel and inspire the light within.

Take time to slow cook foods this week – to sustain you through the week ahead, and to stash in the freezer for when the baby comes.

Journal Prompts

- How can I reclaim a new understanding of slowness this week?
- What areas am I finding most challenging as my pregnancy progresses?
- How can I explore boundaries and balance in relation to each area?

Affirmation: *Slow, still, soft and divinely led I find a new balance.*

Week 24
Prepare for the Best

There appears to be a tendency in humans to think the worst, as if doing so will protect us from pain. I've done it, and I've seen others do it. We look at the array of options and we choose to dwell in the worst possible outcome. In thinking the worst, and exploring it, we trick ourselves that we will be fully prepared when disaster hits.

The problem with this is that the focus on negativity sinks into your bones and becomes a habit. You prepare for one disaster and soon you are inundated with potential turmoil and chaos that you ought to entertain 'just in case'. In being prepared for your nightmares, you are swapping out a life well-lived for existing within the energy of that nightmare daily.

Guess what? You'll never be prepared for every eventuality. The thing you are afraid of will still hurt you, no matter how many preparations you put in place. You will bypass the wonder of life with your eye trained into the dark. Life will become a bleak hole in which you meander and abide.

When my second child's early scan came back full of fear, I lent myself to the abyss for several days. It's a grotesque, dark, saddening place to dwell. I couldn't bear it, this fall into pain. I asked the cosmos for a hand, for some help. At just the moment of asking a lorry drove past me with the word 'HOPE' emblazoned in six-foot writing down the side! Something clicked. I didn't need to prepare for the worst, I could instead swap out the rigours of anxiety for the lightness of hope. In that moment everything changed.

This was profound and has altered my response to difficult times ever since. Hope is one of the most powerful forces I have encountered. Preparing for things we hope for feels thrilling, potent and magical. It lends itself over to manifestation and personal spiritual empowerment in ways that tickle all your senses and change the shape of your life. I am not recommending living in denial of reality or a climate of toxic/false positivity. But looking on the bright side, allowing for the best is just a valid approach as always thinking the worst.

The other thing about preparing for the best, and consciously acting as if all may very well have a good outcome, is that it keeps you calm. It enables you to function and find the joy that exists alongside the worry. And, if indeed the worst does arise, it holds you differently: it buoys you up, it helps you to make empowered decisions and it shoos fear from the room so that every thought and decision is based in love and the next best thing that might happen.

Pregnancy is a dive into deep and divine self-help. Preparing for the best is a potent way to keep your head, hold your course and find an uprising well of inner stillness, even in the most uncertain of situations.

Meditation:
Getting to Know Hope

This meditation ushers you away from the fearful loud voices that can inundate your wellbeing and brings you into alignment with hope. Hope may be a familiar theme, but not something many people often dwell with. Here we give over to the best possibilities and happiest of outcomes, letting yourself really feel into what that might allow.

Take a few deep breaths to settle yourself. Our meditation today is more active and engaging, so it helps to do it sitting up. It calls on you to actively work with your inner experience and shift into a different gear.

Recall a difficult situation, something that you are feeling anxious about. Perhaps start with something minor, like a conversation you need to have or a piece of paperwork you keep putting off. Give yourself a brief overview of this circumstance and acknowledge how it is making you feel. Take note of where this sits in your body, if there is any tension or experiences of sickness, dizziness or unwanted butterflies.

Then with a full intent and understanding that you get to define your experience, shift the storyline of this circumstance. Sit with the very real possibility that this can be dealt with in positive and fulfilling ways. Imagine yourself having dealt with the matter, and it being successfully completed and put behind you. Feel into the liberation and possibility that it will all go well. That no matter what happens, the actioning and processing of the circumstance, will help heal and relieve it. Let hope infuse the situation with possibility.

Ask for the energy of hope to step into your heart and mind. Pray for hope to infiltrate your thoughts and choices. Entertain hope as a very real option.

As the energy for this mediation subsides, bring the possibility of hope with you into the rest of your day, applying it to all things that might usually feel irksome or difficult. As time goes by you may wish to start utilising this energy for bigger life events, and indeed those things that otherwise feel hopeless. For even in the abyss and the darkness of hardships and pain, hope can bring clarity and power that shifts all things.

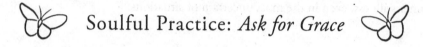

Soulful Practice: *Ask for Grace*

Our prayers are easily made for others, but when was the last time you prayed or dared hope for something you desire? You may have manifestations and dreams you are working towards. This perhaps is the core of your life and attention. Yet, what about the other stuff, the niggly in-between parts of life that are difficult or uncomfortable, the problems you tolerate and the darker aspects of life that have become ordinary and everyday? Have you said a prayer for yourself in relation to these parts lately?

Our Soulful Practice this week is to pinpoint your areas of personal struggle and ask for help. This may be undertaken as a prayer – get on your knees, hands clasped and have a word with your favourite god or goddess. It may also be a more informal conversation you hold with yourself. Openly examining the parts of you that feel tired and wounded, ask your highest self, the forces that be, to give you a helping hand.

In essence you are being asked to 'hand it over', to ask for help and to expect things to shift in more positive directions. I cannot tell you what the result of this will be, only that, in my darkest times, a prayer or a word to some divine something, helps. It helps you to recognise that you are not alone, that there are mysteries of life, invisible yet powerful, who can, when called upon, make magic happen. Even if the miracle you are hoping for doesn't materialise quickly, there is always space and energy for other things to shift, for life to open in surprising ways. Pray, hope and ask for grace for yourself this week, then sit back and allow it to unfold.

Creative Practice: *A Letter of Hope*

Write a letter to yourself, from your future self, and in this letter share all the wonderful things that have happened. This little projection into the future, written to the you of now, will help you to conceive of the best possible path forward. Plus, using your imagination, you can begin to sit with the energies of that beautiful future now. Don't hold back, share this future magic with your current self and give yourself all the hot tips as to how you will make this happen! You can revisit this in a few years' time and begin to witness how some of it may be unfolding!

Journal Prompts

- Do I tend to think the worst or the best of a situation? Where does this tendency come from?

- What situations feel heavy and intolerable to me right now?

- What outcomes might be possible in relation to these difficult situations that feel good, light and positive?

- What is my experience of hope? Is hope something I have actively and consciously worked with before?

- How might my current circumstances work out exceptionally well? – Write this out as if it were already true…

 Affirmation: *I am expecting the best outcome for myself and those I love, in all things.*

Week 25
The Womb is the Safest Space

In our medicalised world it can often feel like your body is a dangerous place to inhabit. We are coming to pregnancy post germ warfare waged by Coronavirus and all the ramifications that this period held for our lives. The limitations and newfound fear around infection are doubtless going to run through your consciousness for decades to come. If you have struggled with pregnancy, endured previous miscarriages, or had problematic periods and related issues such as endometriosis, then pregnancy, combined with all the many risk factors, can feel like a tight-rope walk. Even for those whose pregnancy has come easily and presents no apparent issues, the growing of a baby in our bodies may feel precarious.

There is so much focus on what to do, what not to do, and the pressure to 'count the kicks', that we can become lost in a malaise-like feeling of distrust in our own physical ability. Many of us exist day-to-day, without much thought to how our heart beats, why the skin renews itself or the state of our organs. Our bodies simply exist, suspended by some magic that compels them to live, love and thrive. In pregnancy, however, we become acutely aware of that process and do what we can to support it. This includes entertaining fearful thoughts, so that we might help circumnavigate disaster.

No matter the state of your pregnancy, the warnings you have heard, the potential problems or symptoms that run in the family, it is also true that there is nowhere safer for your baby right now. Let's take that truth as a countenance to any more negative thoughts, allowing the clarity of it to bubble over and above any concern or worries. There simply is nowhere else for the child to be, there is no safety net, no incubator, no cushioned cloud upon which your baby might rest better than they do within your womb. No matter your concerns, real or otherwise, your baby is safest and most beautifully held, precisely where they are.

As we move into the territory of baby's progression, as they protrude further and further into your life, take a moment to recognise that they, in this moment, are exactly and entirely where they should be, and that this place, so loving, so cosy, is the only and the safest place for them.

 Meditation: *Planting a Seed of Clarity*

Lie or sit comfortably, we are creating quiet space for introspection and the clarity of safety within this moment.

Take a few moments with your eyes closed to bring yourself inward. Imagine that your body is a fertile garden, a space of soil and safety. Look to your hands and envision that you are holding a seed, and that this small seed requires to be grown. Recognise that you must place the seed somewhere for this process to begin, and that whilst you may water and nurture it, the life of it happens beyond you. The magic of this is sacred and every day. The reality is that without trust in your inner compost, without being planted, the seed will remain a seed. In your mind's eye, carefully plant the seed into your womb. Utter words of love and lullaby as you cover over this tiny seed, watering it with potential and promise. Take your time here, offer the seed to your inner earth with patience and love.

Breathe deeply into the embedding that you have created. Know that this is all you might do, and that your love and tending is enough. There is nowhere else that this seed may take root, grow and blossom. Allow any loving thoughts or knowing to bubble to the surface.

When you feel fully connected to the seed and the environment you have created, allow yourself to take a deep breath and return to your day. Know that you can return to this seed, the breath and your inner sanctum whenever you feel it necessary.

 Soulful Practice: *Connect with Baby*

I have managed to get to week 25 of this book without suggesting we connect with your baby. It has been important that the focus has been on you, to create a space of health and wellbeing. Now is the time to turn inward, but not to your heart and soul, this week we amp up (or begin) our connection to the child within.

With my first child I nattered away to her from the moment I knew she was present in the womb. I did not shut up, for nine months, playing her music, chattering away. My second and now third child simply didn't receive that same level of vocal activity because, well, life is now so much fuller.

I do still take time to connect. It need not be constant or a thing to tick off on your daily to-do list. Rather, this connection is about seeking out moments of togetherness with your unborn where you bring your energy to them, offer them love in whispers or heartfelt belly-holding. If you have other children or a partner, get them involved, have them whisper or sing or crack jokes at your stomach.

Every so often I love to lie down, place my hands on my belly and wait for the kicks. I take that time to remember what I am brewing and to feel my love expand to the little soul within. I also particularly enjoy the volley of wriggles and kicks I have started to experience at bedtime, not strong enough to wind me or cause discomfort, but little reminders that the babe is here.

Make time and space this week to speak with, sing to, or simply bring your mind and heart to your baby.

Creative Practice:
Creating and Connecting to Your Baby

Spend a moment tuning into your baby. Whilst they are an unknown entity, I believe that we can glean something of their character before birth. I have felt my imagination tune me into aspects of all my children even before I was pregnant with them. A connection that can be explored and mined by your imagination to start to build a picture of parts of who your child might be.

Years before I was pregnant with my first child, I knew her. The closer she came to being, the more my imagination presented her energy, her personality. One day, in a guided shamanic journey before I knew I was pregnant, I envisioned her leap into me like a lion. She certainly holds lioness energy. The next day I took the pregnancy test and bam, there she was.

My second child, a gentler easy-going energy was clear to me for some months before she was conceived. Whilst this third energy, certain to be a boy, one that I was uncertain over for a few years, strode in eventually given a slim opportunity and I have visions of him as a floppy-haired teen, so like this father, and yet not. Each child has shown up through imaginative journeys in my mind, and in some ways, because of this, they feel purposeful, perfect and so very known to me.

We can know our children, as we can source information on anything, with the first powerful port of call being our own inventive minds.

Sit with your child's energy in mind. Call it forward, let what comes be some version of their truth. Write it down, explore it, draw their picture or capture their spirit in poetry, song and art. Brainstorm their attributes, hair colour or potential, allowing your imagination to ramble freely about their persona.

Write a little love letter of hope and joy to your baby. Tell them how you feel about their arrival, about the journey you have been on in growing them, and how you hope to show up for them as a parent. If writing is not your thing, then find ways to express yourself in other ways. You might find a poem you adore and write it out, surrounded by scribbles and pictures, you may wish to start or continue a pregnancy journal that one day you can hand to your child.

 # Journal Prompts

- When I feel my baby move it makes me feel...
- Has your baby moved at a time or in a way that has felt meaningful, perhaps in relation to a name suggestion, or when they have heard a particular sound or voice? Share this...
- How do you intend to be a place of safety for your child, and honour yourself as such, starting now?
- Share all the ways that this pregnancy feels good and right...

 Affirmation: *I am the safest space for my baby to grow*

Week 26
I Don't Wanna!

Humans like to hoard our circumstances. Very few of us are good at letting go of people, places, habits and things. It takes work. Pregnancy (and what comes next) will inundate you with opportunities to release parts of life that no longer serve you, though the trick here is to figure out what those things may be. In the first instance of pregnancy we get rid of the obvious, perhaps that is alcohol, late nights out, caffeine and your love of blue cheese. These changes are as temporary as we want them to be, and of course can be revisited sometime in the future. The change I am talking about here relates to situations more substantial.

For me, at present, it relates to my work. Many of you may be familiar with my work with tarot: I have written books, created card decks, taught tarot and read for thousands of people. At this point in my pregnancy, I just don't really feel like it anymore. I am being pulled in other directions: this book, this baby, potential other explorations of creativity and spirituality, such as oracle cards and women's circles. Whilst I am not rebuking and relenting on tarot (it will always be part of who I am) it's just not something that I feel like spending my time on right now.

This is the measure I want you to use this week. Is there something in your life that you just don't want to do now? Maybe you carry on regardless, doing it anyway. Deep down, you'd rather not because it doesn't feel as natural or easy as it used to. How is this inner inclination of teenage 'I don't wanna!' trying to tell you something? I have other objections too: my achy hips are lining up with my mind and both are complaining about the cleaning: 'I don't wanna!' Similarly, the daily dog walking, something I have found such solace in for years, has been drawn into the field of 'urgh, but do I have to?'

We may beat ourselves up for this, thinking we are becoming lazy or discontent. The truth is, some awkward (yet wise) inner voice is rebelling. There is a chance here to rejig the status quo, to draw new lines in the sand, and to see what the clearing of space brings to the surface.

Step fully into your 'I don't wanna!' this week and see where it leads. If you don't fancy a job, task or opportunity, then simply don't. Allow yourself space to create a big fat 'no' and express it as you take pressure off and begin to embrace the inner teenage 'nah!'.

 # Meditation: *Inner Rebel*

Within this meditation we will pull on the rebellious teenage energy buried within. Whether this was something you experienced in your teens, or repressed in some way, this is an opportunity to meet and greet the vitality and creativity of spunky adolescent attitude.

This meditation might be best played out with the accompaniment of some of your teenage kicks, perhaps youthful music playing in the background. If there was a band or singer that triggered your teenage angst and helped you to feel more like yourself, then play that on a loop whilst undertaking this session.

As you sit and breathe, gently close your eyes and in your mind's eye take yourself to a safe and wonderful place from your teenage years. It could be your bedroom, a classroom, a friend's house, or if you can't find a suitable place, create a mental image of somewhere your inner teen would have felt safe and held.

Ask your inner teenager to step forward and sit with you. No matter your age, (and I appreciate some readers may still be in their teens), the part of yourself you are addressing is the energy of youth. Not the spirit of your childlike self, but rather, the character and persona of you as you transitioned from childhood to adulthood. Each person's teen is likely to be quite different, and in this space, I encourage you to meld with their unique energy, to listen to their feelings, and to honour their thoughts and feelings as they arise in this moment.

What does your teenage energy have to say to you? How would it like to feel seen and witnessed? How can it infuse with your current situations and allow for growth and expansion?

As the meditation wanes, bring your heart and hands together with your teen, offer love and promises of protection and care. Let this inner aspect of yourself know that they can and will be heard throughout your life. Imagine making space for her to sit within your inner council of wisdom.

When you are ready, return to the room.

Soulful Practice:
Treat Your Angst Right

Take your inner angsty 'can't be bothered' teenager out for a walk. This may be around your local area, or further afield into a city or town. Visit the places she would have liked and appreciated and do whatever the heck she'd love to do. This may show up in many ways, as per the individual, what matters is that you tune into the persona of your inner rebellious youngster and take her to do whatever she likes!

Creative Practice:
Destruction to Create

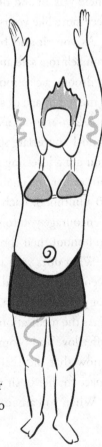

Teenage energy is stereotypically quite destructive. Interestingly this often leads to some of the world's most profound creations. Teenage angst is responsible for so much incredible music, art, business ideas and writing. Adolescents want to make the world their own, and don't like much direction from those who believe themselves older and wiser. Disrupt, interrupt, change things up this week... Below are a few ideas to channel teenage creation into your life this week.

I encourage you to call the power of destruction into your creativity this week. It may involve scrapping or reworking something you are working on violently, or with a carefree attitude and with disregard to any intention. Watch and see if the absence of concern about the outcome of your creation allows for a more liberated approach.

- Let loose with your boundaries and write, sing, create, move and present yourself in ways outside of the usual grown-up box. Channel your era and the styles of your adolescent times and let this walk you differently into every room.

- Graffiti the sidewalk with chalk, writing messages of empowerment and glee for others to stumble on. Carve your initials into a tree or a fence in some far-flung field.

- Write a poem all about how you feel and make it as heartfelt and soul-led as possible without querying what would happen if someone read it.

- Have your 'Dear Diary' moment and let loose with all your hopes, desires and moaning to paper, in the way only a 15-year-old can.

- Lock yourself away, lie about without a screen to distract you and play your favourite tracks from your teenage playlist, as loud as you feel comfortable.

 ## Journal Prompts

- Who was my teenage self? Describe their hopes desires and plans.

- What did my inner teenager care about most of all?

- How did she feel empowered and disempowered? How does some of this carry through to today?

- If your teenage self could speak to you now, what would she say?

- What would you say back?

 Affirmation: *I connect to all energies within me and trust them to offer wisdom and guidance.*

Week 27
The Wisdom of Others

For much of this book we are focusing on the wisdom within us, giving ourselves permission to feel into what is right for ourselves. This week, however, we are practicing the art of asking for help, the magic of sourcing wisdom and information from another trusted person or group that hold answers we do not ourselves have yet.

Instinct and intuition are vital to pregnancy, parenthood and life, though it cannot be done in a vacuum, as they say, it takes a village. At times we need to outsource to those who can help hold and sustain us. Such people and organisations can fall into many categories, depending on what it is you seek. The admission here is that we cannot go at life alone, and that there are times when we may need to expand our knowledge with the assistance of others. Such others may be trusted friends and family, or experts and wisdom keepers such as your therapist, doctor, mentor, midwife, governmental body, astrologer, cleaner or acupuncturist. The types of support and assistance needed and those who offer it are incredibly diverse. It is in the hands of these folks, be they masseuses or professors, that we find what we need at any given moment.

My need this week was prompted by severely aching hips. I needed help with the cleaning. Such a simple thing, yet I carried on mopping like a good martyr and then suffering as a result. In the end I asked a friend, who is also a cleaner, to come and help me out every so often, for the time being. It changed everything. In other areas of need, I asked my husband to put his foot down at work and not to work away anymore. He has been far from home for eight weeks, whilst I would usually crack on resiliently, I have had to recognise that I'm physically and emotionally struggling with the load. Last night, I asked my mum, visiting for two days, to have my kids so I could write and edit this book in the evening: need met.

Take time this week to consider where you may need to request help or guidance. Allowing yourself to reach out and be held is beautifully connective, and connection is a source of power and inspiration that can elevate you to greater heights. There is no shame in wanting to be better, to know more, or to have your hand held. Let your needs be met by those who hold the key to your current issues and problems.

Meditation: *Spiritual Help*

This meditation will be focused on actively seeking spiritual help and support. Please be open to this and cast it in a light that feels comfortable. The source we are accessing is a wondrous, connective and loving universal one, this may be god, spirit, angels or perhaps some other higher source you feel comfortable with.

Take a deep breath, close your eyes and come to resting. Imagine that you are sat or lying upon a cloud. This cloud is floating safely and peacefully above the Earth. You are elevated and floating above all your everyday worries, gaining a much larger perspective on life and your current circumstances.

The cloud starts to rise higher, taking you into the cosmos and the heavens. It is stunningly beautiful, surrounded by stars, lights and colours. Allow yourself to give over to this ride, knowing you are safe and protected. The cloud carries you to a space that feels familiar, you disembark and find an ornate chair with your name on it. There is another chair beside you. It is time to invite and welcome in a cosmic guide, ancestor or angelic helper. Call gently for help and watch as a wiser loving being arrives to sit with you.

This is your time with your guide, god, ancestor, angel or aspect of your highest self to take a moment to connect, ask questions or share your worries. Allow the spirit visiting you to listen and respond in a way that feels deeply comforting. Take heed and feel into how they gift you words, wisdom or new feelings. Continue to sit and converse with this glorious aspect of your divine connected self until such time as the moment naturally ends.

As it does so, thank your helper and return to your cloud, where you are slowly and safely brought back to Earth. Take a deep breath, wiggle your fingers and toes and return to the room. You may find it helpful to journal about any images, feelings or words you received within this meditation.

Soulful Practice: *Surrender*

Surrender does not mean giving up, not in this instance. Rather, it means that it is time to give over to your current reality. Maybe you cannot be in control of everything. Perhaps you cannot cope anymore with certain things. Possibly you need to talk something through, or it might be you just need a helping hand and a back rub. Whatever it is you surrender to, do so purposefully and consciously. It is good to recognise that you require others, and that they can offer you kindness and solutions.

Allow yourself to be in a place of need. Know that sometimes the only way to cope, expand or grow, is by being in that need, and receiving something that is necessary. Need is important. Plants need earth, light and water. Being deprived of those things causes wilting and hardship. You too have needs and you cannot meet them all yourself. Surrender to your needs, let them speak, allow them to find answers in the hands and hearts of others.

 ## Creative Practice: *Creative Surrender*

Often when we start a creative project, we have an idea of what we want it to look, feel or taste like. As you embark on your Creative Practice this week, I challenge you to surrender. Trust the process that arises and to move into your creation without any expectations of what it is you are creating. Take the pressure off yourself to perform, or to make a certain something. Creation for its own sake, as children recognise, is an adventure enough. Let your creativity this week be liberated by the possibility that it need not mean a thing, that it isn't serious and that you don't need to advertise or monetise it. Get back to grass roots, surrender to the process of creating, without a view as to what that should become.

Instead of feeling your creativity must always stem from you, why not lean into the expertise of others this week: follow an online tutorial, a recipe or guidebook, learn a skill from a friend, ask a family member for practical help with a current creative project, for their feedback.

 ## Journal Prompts

- What area(s) of life am I finding particularly tricky? Who may I source to assist me with this?

- How do I feel about being assisted?

- How might I feel on the other side of having been helped?

 Affirmation: *I allow myself to be carefully held and helped.*

THIRD
TRIMESTER

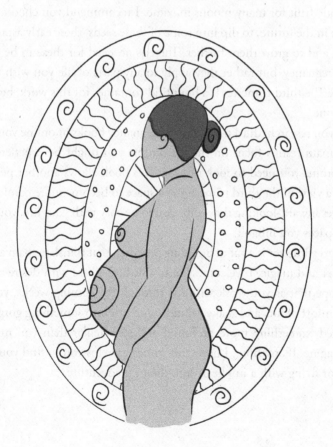

The third trimester begins at week twenty-eight and represents the final weeks of your pregnancy. This last trimester sees your child tripling in weight and your bump expanding significantly. This time and space may feel physically restrictive, as you grapple with your expanding body and the host of issues this may create.

In other ways, this trimester is elevating and liberating. It is, I believe, an opportunity to go deeper into who you are becoming, to explore your craft more deeply, and adventure further into your soulful expression and your creativity. Where the physical cannot go, the heart and spirit do not fear to tread. This last leg of pregnancy is a testament to evolving into a more rounded soul, one who is ready for the road that lies ahead, who has tools in their well woven basket and is prepared for the shifts and changes that the coming months and years promise to provide.

Many of the themes from week 28 onwards are huge, spirited life lessons. They carry with them seeds of potential which you can start to plant now, but that will provide fruit for many moons to come. I recommend you choose to revisit this book in the future, to dip into some of these seeds, these early aspirations of your life, and to grow them further. There is no need for these to be beholden only to pregnancy, but rather they apply to any parts of life you wish to gestate and grow. The third trimester is a bountiful container for this work, but it is not the only one.

When you research 'third trimester' in pregnancy books or online you will find that the main results focus on the discomfort you might be experiencing and the symptoms you need to look out for. This book allows another perspective. It fosters a view of the third trimester as a space to become more comfortable. It encourages inward-looking that helps you to be cosy with your life, your choices and the spaces you inhabit.

The third trimester is a vat of bubbling potential that translates pain and worry into power and magic. I welcome you to this next phase with desire and abandon. I hope that as you work with me through the coming weeks, you loosen the discomfort of life, and shake, shudder and roll into something gorgeous and unexpected, something more profound and spectacular than you might have dared imagine. If anything, I hope this trimester helps you to find yourself, just in time for flying with a full heart into the next adventure.

Week 28
Legacy

We are the bridges to our babies' lives. Some of the legacy we will pass down to our children is biological, some cultural: DNA, character traits, illnesses, talents, physical characteristics, patterns of behaviour… Our family and cultural legacy travel through us, sometimes skipping generations, sometimes coming through when we least expect them. Some of our legacy gets passed on automatically, but much of this we get to choose.

We might have issues with the ways we were raised: minor and major issues, through to full on trauma. The past can be a difficult place to navigate: it can leave us feeling ill at ease as to how we might change legacies, break curses, and start anew. Contemplating our legacy is something we might want to put off worrying about till later… Yet here we are embarking on it though our cells, blood, joints and bones: it is happening right now.

I didn't think much about my legacy with my first or second child, I just wanted to be the best mother I possibly could be. I took all the brilliant parts of my own childhood and amplified them, creating a home filed with creativity, animals and as much nature as the kids can stomach. I parented as I would have wished to have been parented and emulated the better parts of my own parents' legacies.

I enjoyed sharing what was magical to me with my brood and felt grateful that I too had experienced it. I was lucky enough to have living grandparents, and spaces that I had grown up in still in existence, I took my children there often, as it felt deeply important to pass them on whilst I could.

At my grandmother's recent memorial, my aunt gave a beautiful speech about how she and my father had been raised. I realised that the way I live now, is part of my grandmother's legacy. And here I was thinking I had conjured this approach all by myself!

At some point though there is a fracture, a point when what you have previously known reaches its limits, and you are left with space. A space in which to create a new legacy, to do things differently. The opportunity to follow a path you haven't yourself walked. You could shy back into the familiar, or expand yourself, for the benefit of your kids and your family: to do things differently. This might involve sharing in a partner's skills or loves, or things they did with their family that feel alien to you. It may also be that you have outgrown the old and are ready for a blast of something entirely new. This is evolution, and experienced healthily and with love at its centre, you start to create a new legacy.

Of course, some of you may be reading this with naught but difficult memories of your own childhood. If this is you, then you get to create. You can collage an amalgamation of what it is to be a good parent or carer, without ever having experienced it. You can identify what you will not do and consider what the opposite might be. You can think on what your inner child needed and make that your focus and priority. You can source books, films, historical characters, wise mentors and long forgotten moments of kindness for the seeds of what you may bring forward. In how you respond to your legacy, you have a blank slate and you hold the chalk.

Parenting has made me deeply grateful for my own parents and what they brought to the table, though at times I see their shortcomings more sharply, as I know they saw their parents' too. We have the privilege of doing things differently, yet potentially still making mistakes. We will do things we regret. We will face unprecedented times and unique circumstances. How we handle these and how we move forward is the measure of our mothering.

There is no real answer here, it's all rather philosophical, particularly as the moment tends to sweep us away abruptly. This week, and in the time before baby is born, is a time to contemplate who you are becoming, how you might make a legacy of this new relationship. All great revolutions start within, with an idea, or a hope. What is yours?

Meditation

"I am the beginning of a new line, all good things come through me, I trust and empower my choices and my actions."

Take these words into a simple meditation practice this week. Let them infuse with your hopes and desires and allow whatever bubbles within to find its way to the surface. Breathe deeply into these words, and the unique meaning they hold for you. Allow yourself to journal upon what comes up for you as you focus on this simple mantra.

Soulful Practice:
Plant a Legacy Houseplant

My grandmother's Christmas cactus blossoms wildly on my bathroom window ledge as I type this. It is bright orange and glorious. The first buds started to arrive the week of her memorial and have continued to light up that space for weeks now. Another cactus of hers sits on my kitchen windowsill and her photo on my shelf. There is something quite wonderful about owning a piece of something living that she was invested in. Much like me, I too am something she was invested in. There is legacy right here, in the watering, the trust, the keeping alive of her spirit.

Choose a plant that breeds itself and allows for babies and future growth. Cacti and succulents are a good choice for indoor plants, and they need little watering and attention (an important consideration with baby on the way!). Or plant something outside: nasturtiums, lupins and calendula are all self-seeding and give beautiful bright flowers year after year. Dedicate the plant to your lineage. Re-pot it and devote yourself to its care. As you nurture and look after this small living being, trust that it might outlive you, that some part of it could end up in your great grandchild's home or garden.

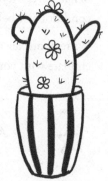

Creative Practice: *Legacy Creation*

Think on the type of ancestor that you hope to be. It is easy to feel disconnected from the generations that follow you. There may be clear bonds between you and your future grandchildren and great-grandchildren. Beyond that it may be hard to envisage. Yet it is those future humans that will carry parts of your energy and dynamism into the next era, perhaps living the dreams you were unable to make space for.

With a future generation in mind, think on how you might communicate with this future collection of people. What do you wish for them? How does this reflect what you wish for yourself and your children in this very moment? What actions may you take now to be an inspiration for those future people? How might your blockages, overcome by you in this lifetime, clear passageways for your great-great-grandchildren to be greater? Envision the very best for their future, and pull this energy into the present, for this is where it begins. You may wish to write a letter, plant a tree, create an image, crochet a blanket with the meaning of your prayers to the future imbued within it.

Journal Prompts

- What aspects of your childhood, even small fragments of memories, give you a steer and a lead into what you might like to bring to your parental legacy?

- How do you feel about the way you were parented? What would you do differently/the same?

- What parts of your legacy are you worried about? (This might be health conditions or behaviours that are prevalent in your family.)

- Write about an important experience you have had that you would like to emulate with your legacy.

 Affirmation: *I trust my ability to create a wonderful legacy.*

Week 29
Loss and Grief

Pregnancy may cocoon our child from the harsh realities of life, yet it does not offer us the same protection. Loss and grief can visit us more poignantly as we sit with this other end of the spectrum of life-giving. Your feelings related to these subjects may not hang around a specific event, nobody need become ill or die for a response to loss and death to be awoken. Indeed, the very nature of our world, what we see on the news, a video we catch in brief online or a conversation with a friend may be a catalyst to some bout of deep inner mourning.

Bringing a child into a world so beset with troubles, so inundated with fear and with an awareness that their bright light will one day succumb to illness and death is a reality of pregnancy. It is a reality of pregnancy that has us feeling depths of mind-numbing sadness, that goes beyond fear for our own lives.

Death is the other end of the spectrum, and yet it can feel chillingly close. My current pregnancy started with death, with the loss of my grandma. Since then my other grandma has given us quite a few scares, our parents have gotten older, their abilities change, my mother-in-law has succumbed far too young to the later stages of dementia and several people in my awareness have become visibly older and sicker. There is no respite from the realities of our world, though a babe in body and arms is one short-lived way to hold a middle finger to the inevitable.

You may encounter events during this time that bring you up close and personal to loss, grief, pain, sickness and death. You may experience them personally as you move through your nine months, with actual loss and shifts in wellness of those you love. You may simply become deeply empathic and tearful when stories of such things head your way.

The beauty of the cycles of life are not without huge spikes and barbs of suffering. We grow babies and give birth in the knowledge that one day, we then they, will leave this Earth. I have found that this interminable wheel of life is only ever made easier by my spiritual faith. It is from within a belief in 'something more' that endings are softened, and illness takes different shapes. This is not to say that we should circumnavigate our pain, but rather, absorb it into a wider view, one that holds hope for life continuing onwards, in some unknown, celestial or inspired new form.

As you are here, I assume you have an open heart towards a spiritual path. Sitting with pain, in the face of new life, is an exquisite contradiction, one of bounty and frustratingly inarguable unfairness. It is in this space that I find comfort in the grey area, in the magic that has arisen in my own life. I remember those moments I have felt departed loved ones draw near, and the never-ending accuracy of my tarot cards that seems to be a hint towards a greater power.

This week we wade into the depths of grief and our fear of death and from this space find a place where we might acknowledge our inner desire for celestial comfort. In this dark estranged place, we may conjure greater understandings of an evermore, a belief system or a powerful inner charge that lets us know that death and moments of intense pain are simply not, and never were, the end.

 ## Meditation: *Touching the Cosmic*

This meditation takes the concept of divinity, of the sacred, the unknown and allows you to meet and touch it. Give yourself a good half hour or so to unfurl into this medicinal and healing session.

You may wish to accompany this meditation with some spiritual work and practice. If you have a deck of tarot or oracle cards, take a moment to connect with them and pull a card. Allow this to be your guide and entry point as you take the energy of what it brings into your meditation. You may also like to hold a favourite crystal or even a flower, rock or piece of special jewellery as touch-point within the meditation.

Moving into relaxation in our usual way, hand on heart, take three deep breaths.

We move into this meditation with a goal to meet with some cosmic part of ourselves, or a loving entity that exists beside us – take whichever feels more comfortable.

In your imagination bring yourself into a cocoon of spirit, allow a cosmic egg of swirling energy to surround you. This is your sacred space; you are safe and protected here. Breathe into the deep and healing energies that swirl around you and trust that they are all here for your benefit in this lifetime. When you feel ready usher an invitation to the 'cosmic'. You may say the following words in your mind or aloud:

"I welcome connection with a loving cosmic force who has wisdom, lessons and power for me."

Lie back and be with the moment. Be in the peace of your swirling cosmic safe space. Let thoughts arise and pass. Witness the feelings, understandings and visuals that arise. You may feel or hear messages that feel pertinent and inspiring. You may simply enjoy a mind show of patterns and colours that feels imaginary – but remember imagination is a tool of the divine.

You may also use this space and moment with the divine to ask for healing, to offer prayers for self and others or to gently connect with the highest intent that the universe holds for you at this moment. Breathe into all of this and pull the cosmic internally, trusting that the energies you welcome in will continue to work with you for time to come, helping you to grow.

Stay with this cosmic intent if it feels comfortable. When you are ready thank the energy and bring yourself to an awareness of the room. Breath and wiggle to reenergise, open your eyes and lie for a little while before moving back to the rest of your day.

Soulful Practice:
Examining Your Evidence

In the face of loss and grief it is natural to succumb to darker feelings, numbness and a sense of abiding nothingness. This is something to honour and sit with, to experience the depths life offers. Within these most difficult of emotions there is space for a chink of light, of hope, and this can be found by exploring and acknowledging your own personal evidence that there is 'something more' beyond the life we currently live.

My spiritual path has always had me examining life in alternative ways. I have found that people who are not even especially spiritual have a little collection of heart-warming anecdotes regarding magical things that have happened to them that defy explanation. These stories collect in our consciousness and help us to attribute some meaning to death, sickness and horror that suggests that there is wonder and connection that occurs even once the body has died.

At a funeral recently my uncle spoke about how when he attended the funeral of a young friend who died many years ago, a shaft of light appeared from nowhere to hit the coffin. As it did so a butterfly flew up and followed the shaft of light into the sky. My uncle reported this with some cynicism, but the fact he had held the story and shared it all these years later showed that whatever he chose to tell himself about the incident, it was in some way meaningful to him and others who had needed a magical connection at that time.

Many other people have shared experiences with me, almost embarrassed by saying them out loud. The time they felt their mother draw close after she died, the bugs, birds, rainbows and butterflies that took them by surprise in meaningful ways and pertinent times of grief, the electronics that go crazy upon death despite having no batteries or not being plugged in. The stories are endless. We witness them, and then we bury them, for they don't sit well with a more scientific or logical approach. Occasionally we may get these memories out and dust them off, only to quickly shuffle them off again to focus on 'real life'.

There does seem to be a mass collection of evidence that many people keep secret. When we examine this personal evidence it presents a picture, often one that is quite compelling. Maybe we are looking for solution and salve or perhaps, from some sacred space, that solution and salve is finding us...

Your Soulful Practice this week is to contemplate your evidence. Write it down, make it real, talk about it with a loving and like-minded friend. Hold it up to the light and allow it to breathe. This is your personal collection of the extraordinary. You don't need to make sense of it or talk it into nothingness. It happened, you experienced it, let it be a real thing, let it be known even if only to yourself.

 Creative Practice: *Honouring Life*

I can't take grief and loss out of the equation of pregnancy or life. The tricky nature of existence is beyond us both. Yet we can find ways to celebrate the life we find ourselves within, no matter how precarious or sticky that may be. Our conscious creative task this week is to create a celebration of life. I love the idea of a collage, or a mess of paint, perhaps a soul deep exploration of words and music to counter pain and uplift. Ideas of what you could create are:

- A beautiful vase of flowers that brings the colours of the season and vibrates powerfully to remind us of the blossoming of life, that moment we sit thankfully within.

- Throw colours at a canvas that feel rainbow bright and childlike. Give yourself permission to be wild and reckless.

- Create an affirming playlist of songs that honour all things celebratory, listen to it on a loop and whenever mood elevation is required.

- Write about your happiest memories and lose yourself in the feelings, smells and depths of them.

- Visit a gallery or museum and observe the human spirit in all its imaginative, creative and scientific glory.

Journal Prompts

- What griefs and losses have I experienced in recent times? Write about them and speak about the contradictions and thoughts this raises as you prepare to birth life...

- I have experienced the supernatural or unexplainable in the following ways...

- How might my spirituality and belief systems support me now?

Affirmation: *I exist beyond the obvious.*
Loss and grief are necessary shades within my
palette of life learning and experience.

Week 30
Body Love

Three quarters of the way through your pregnancy and the kicks of baby are becoming quite the reality! Your body is changing continuously, and life might feel very different. You may be raring to claim your body back, or you could be lost to the magic of the inner gestation. You sit on the precipice of all kinds of expansion and are likely still just as bustling and busy as ever.

I have two crosses to bear in relation to pregnancy and the way it makes you public property. The first I spoke about earlier, referencing the comments I had suffered under when revealing my pregnancy early on. More recently, I have had the dubious joy of folks commenting on my body. Something which for some reason in pregnancy seems to be fair game.

My body, like your body, is private. The changes we live through as we grow a child are intense and can feel wounding as our known self gives way to something other. Having the opinions or insecurities of others projected onto our physical frames at this time (or any time) can be deeply challenging.

Mostly the challenge is because the projections of others tend to reflect our own bodily issues. It can feel like a real emotional tinderbox that could go up at any moment. The loss of familiarity with weight gain, bust size, skin tone and what may occur during birthing can be a place of real anxiety.

Plus, unhelpfully, we are all subjected to images of women snapping back into shape in the media and online. There is such a weight placed on pregnancy to 'leave no marks', fuelling big business in stretch mark cream during pregnancy, and body-shaping underwear and workout classes for post-birth bodies. But pregnancy inevitably will leave our bodies changed. In fact, it would be strange if such a momentous physical and spiritual event left us unchanged.

This week our work is to sit with the potential of bodily change and recognise that this too is a rite of passage, and a moment in which we can truly choose self-love over and above the painful flagellations of anybody else's gaze or expectations.

The body is a miracle, everybody's body, no matter the gender, age or ability. The idea of body judgment is one truly powerful way to keep you in your place, to have you regretting your every action. The opposite of such judgment is freedom, liberation and power in choosing to view the body as tool of life, experience and expression. The body is a home within which we live it all. We can choose that living to be peppered with nasty or downcast opinions or we can evolve and let the body be host to magic, miracle and beautiful happenings.

It can, of course, take some work and effort to slough off the old and outdated feelings we have about our physicality, especially at such a tender time. Yet it is that tenderness, the magic of the moment, the birthing of self and baby that ultimately demands we do just that. There is space here to acknowledge how we hurt or to admit to the fears we may have regarding our physical being. Equally, there is space to begin to overcome all of that, to hold the body as sacred, and to recognise it as a force of nature that enables you but does not ever truly define you.

 ## Meditation: *Body as Home*

Bring yourself into comfort and relaxation. You may wish to take a bath, sit in nature, or enjoy a warm shower as you undertake this. Hold your hands over any physical spaces that feel tricky or challenged at this moment. If you can't reach them, envision them, and hold them in your heart.

Bring yourself to these words:

"This moment of physical change is necessary and empowering; I offer love to the aspects of myself that are shifting to accommodate this birth."

Close your eyes. Be in your body, stroke, hold, hug yourself, and bring yourself to these words repeatedly. Let words of appreciation and gratitude for your body's work bubble to the surface if they wish. Give over to relaxation whilst leaning into a few moments of self-love. Let your body rest as you see her in her wholeness and ability. Conjure gratitude for all that your body is allowing and thanks for the miracles she enables. Be with this appreciation as you fall into peacefulness, or maybe even allow yourself to nap.

Repeat this meditation daily, maybe several times a day. Tune into the energy of bodily gratitude to help overcome any more negative or tricky feelings.

Soulful Practice:
Body as Altar to Be Adorned and Worshipped

Your body is a mammalian creature that requires belonging, nourishment and safety. It is also a place of cultural expression and a space to source devout faith in your beliefs. This week our Soulful Practice is to move beyond the physical needs of our body, and shift into how your body might tell a story. The body is a canvas that writes its own imaginative truth, but that also submits to adornment of that truth.

This week I encourage you celebrate your physical self as it is now. Adorn it. Express yourself in ways that help you to feel different to how you felt before. Give yourself the gift of external decoration. As shallow as this might sound, there is magic woven into the presentation we choose to shroud ourselves in, and a small shift here or there can conjure courage, self-awareness and confidence.

Perhaps this is the week you finally get that haircut, wear your grandmother's ring, or dig out that spectacular pair of maternity trousers you've been saving for the right moment. If you enjoy make up then perhaps some exploration can be done here, conjuring a new look, or using a slick of gloss or eye dust to bring yourself out of the passive into the present. You may like to pop a few crystals in your pockets or wear the funkiest pair of socks anyone ever did see.

Make yourself feel fully present as you are, in whatever way works: bright colours, flower in your hair or a spritz of something delicious smelling on your clothing. It's all up for grabs, allow yourself to be a conduit of joy, colour or life-giving style.

As you present yourself in your own quirky ways, allow this presentation to echo something of your heart and soul. A reminder that life goes on through this maternal moment, and that the essence of you is articulated not just through flesh, but can be found within your creative, soulful illustration of self.

Creative Practice: *Bump Images*

Whilst on one hand we are dressing our bodies and bumps to be a representation of your inner world, we are also going to get quite vulnerable and raw with our naked bodies. We are not here for hiding or distracting, but in our creativity, we are working to celebrate the parts of us that are changing.

This week's focus is on your ever-expanding bump. Your challenge is to record your bump in some way that is joyful and meaningful to you. Ideas include:

- **Paint** – cover your bump in non-toxic paint or face paint and print with it onto paper as a beautiful colourful keepsake. Or use body paints or henna to decorate your bump. If you have children in your life, let them go wild with your body as canvas.

- **Photo** – photograph your bump in interesting ways: holding flowers, with your body beautifully draped or with intriguing lighting that creates shadows and mystery.

- **Cast** – if you have the energy or wherewithal, you might find a local service that creates a plaster cast of your stomach. Have this done and keep it as an art piece, covered with your scribbles and colourful paint.

- **Clay** – grab some clay or make your own salt dough (one part salt, one part flour, one part hot water and mix till the consistency is doughy – adding flour/water as needed) and have a go at re-creating a mini-me version of your pregnant self and decorating it as you wish.

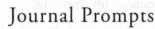

Journal Prompts

- How would I describe my relationship with my body prior to pregnancy?

- How has this shifted during this pregnancy, and what am I experiencing now?

- How have I punished my body in the past? How might I make up for these punishments?

- What amazing and memorable experiences has my body allowed me to have?

- How can I best support my physical self in all healing, energy raising and future magical and creative pursuits?

 Affirmation: *My body is a vessel of passion, creation and expression, I honour all my body's needs and desires.*

Week 31

Developing Deeper Connection

This week is all about developing greater connection – to our energetic selves, our spiritual selves and our creative selves. These final weeks of pregnancy, we are energetically open, more than at any other times at our lives, so this is the natural time to really connect with these aspects of ourselves and our abilities with ease and joy.

There may be experiences during these later weeks that feel psychic in nature, or at least deeply intuitive and instinctive. In this pregnancy I have been much more connected to the intent and feelings of other people. This has taken many different forms.

- Compassion for those in pain and suffering.

- Empathy to people in difficult life situations.

- Exhaustion from hectic and ungrounded interactions with certain folk.

- Urgency and threat that had me leave the local park when a nearby man had me feeling deeply uncomfortable (despite it being broad daylight and plenty of people around).

- Emotionality around my own experiences and deep bouts of tearfulness as feelings flood through me relating to anything, everything, and all parts of my forty-four-year existence on planet Earth.

This deep dive into personal feeling and diverse connection to others has been overwhelming at times, though I do believe it to be part of the process of becoming more connected with who I am and what I need to recognise at any given moment.

This week we will ride the events that come with an understanding that divine connection comes in many ways, and that the ability to read the meaning to every happening lies energetically within – we are the guru able and ready to start to understand the messages and connections that we contain and experience – all by ourselves.

We will also explore the chakras in the meditation. Chakras are the ancient Indian system for understanding our spiritual energy. We will work on clarifying these parts of our bodies so we can prepare for seer-like insight now and in all things moving forward. As we cleanse and clear our chakras and energetic bodies, we make space for communication from our spiritual self, which is really the goal of the deep connection we wish to create.

 # Meditation: *Chakras*

Take a deep breath and allow yourself to relax and get out of your own way for a few minutes. Imagine a sacred light surrounding you like a bubble, keeping you safe as you undertake this connection to spirit.

We will begin by breathing into your chakra points, creating clarity and ease in these spaces and removing any blockages.

As you sit within your bubble of protective energy, bring your attention to each point that I direct and imagine the light of the bubble to move to this point, bringing with it healing and empowerment.

The base chakra is located at base of your spine and is the energetic space that holds your connection to earth, to your grounding and connection to self. Envision a bright red portal or flower opening. Imagine all the healing spiritual energy flowing in and helping to remove unwanted energies and blockages. Ask for grounding, healing and connection as the energies move up through this chakra.

The sacral chakra is located at your perineum between your legs, reaching your sexual organs and womb, fuelling these spaces with fertility, energy and surprising spirituality and intuition (remember those sexual knowings or attractions that seem to stem from this clear and vibrating intelligent part of yourself). Envision a vibrant orange portal or flower opening and all the healing spiritual energy flowing in and helping to remove unwanted energies and blockages. Ask for balance, release, healing of sexual wounds and the heightening of fertility and sacred power.

The solar plexus chakra is located at your solar plexus, the space in your lower middle chest/upper stomach where your ribs meet below your heart and lungs. This place holds your source of personal power and will. Envision a beautiful yellow portal or flower opening. Imagine all the healing spiritual energy flowing in and helping to remove unwanted energies and blockages. Ask for the removal of blocks to your intuition and instinct, the release of any stored anxiety and fear.

The heart chakra is located in the centre of your chest. The heart chakra contains your emotional intelligence, love and deep personal and psychic knowing. Envision a glowing green portal or flower opening and all of the healing spiritual energy flowing into your heart and body, and helping to remove unwanted energies and blockages. Request the energy to heal any old, fractured wounds, any pain of loss, rejection, grief and sadness. Ask for your heart to be made whole and to enable access of the intelligence within this space.

The throat chakra is located in the centre of your throat. Here we find our ability to express, to communicate and to connect to truth. Envision a light turquoise blue portal or flower opening and all the healing spiritual energy flowing in and helping to remove unwanted energies and blockages. Ask that healing is brought to things said and unsaid, that the energy allows for truth to be spoken and clarity to be emanated easily.

The third eye chakra is located in the centre of your forehead. This chakra governs your subtle interactions with your world including the spiritual and intuitive. Envision a deep blue portal or flower opening and all the healing spiritual energy flowing in and helping to remove unwanted energies and blockages. Ask for this space to be cleansed and cleared of anxiety or overthinking, allowing for clear sight and true spirited understandings.

The crown chakra is located just above the crown of the head – this is a spiritual portal allowing direct contact with the divine and enabling wisdom beyond yourself. Envision a rich violet portal or flower opening and all the healing spiritual energy flowing in and helping to remove unwanted energies and blockages. Request blocks to your spiritual power and connection to be removed and to create a steady flow of connection with the divine in the highest possible ways.

Sitting now with all chakras blessed and purified, imaging the light to be infiltrating your body and swirling all around. Take a moment to ask for spiritual connection, welcoming it into your everyday in easy, clear ways.

"I welcome the spiritual within my life, I trust the spiritual to connect with me in ways that are uplifting and empowering, I welcome my spiritual connection."

Pause and sit with this for some time.

When you are ready, imagine there is a little cloud overhead and it begins to rain silver rain down on you. This closes the open chakras to the appropriate degree (the chakra houses its own intelligence and control over this) and helps wash away any residual toxicity and difficulty. Breathe deeply and allow the transformative energy to ebb away before returning to the room.

Soulful Practice:
A Reading to Divine Your Family

I use tarot cards and oracle cards often to divine a loving and empowering reflection of where I am in life at any given moment. The tarot cards work in tandem with my imagination and intuition to present guidance, meaningful messages and imagery. For me the cards are about life creation and not prediction, using them for reflection is a powerhouse of self-realisation and in time personal change and growth (check out my book *Dirty & Divine* or my deck *Rebel Heart Tarot* to explore this gently). You can also use runes, oracle cards or any other divination tool that you find intriguing. This exercise may be most powerful to undertake alongside the week's meditation.

Bring yourself to your tool or your cards, feel them in your hands, and ask for protection and wise insight from the sacred.

You will then pull three cards that will reflect on the following situations:

Card 1 – What your pregnancy is teaching you about your spirituality.

Card 2 – What the connection to your unborn child is bringing to your life from a divine and soulful perspective.

Card 3 – How can you choose to learn and grow because of this spiritual new dawn of pregnancy, birth and parenthood.

Sit with these cards for a while, perhaps making notes or researching the meaning you find upon them.

Finally, pick one more card – this is a wild card. Ask the universe to simply present you with one more thing you need to know about your spiritual path at this moment. Let the card speak and allow yourself time to reflect.

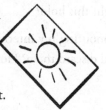 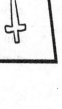

Creative Practice: *Colourful Connection*

This week's Creative Practice is dedicated to colour. Colour is one of the easiest ways we can engage with unseen energies and shift them in our favour.

- You might find you are drawn to certain chakras in the meditation. Perhaps you would like to wear this colour, or sew, knit or crochet something featuring this colour.

• Draw or paint an image of your energy body as you experience it now – using the colours of the chakras or your aura.

• See if you are drawn to creating something in a new colour palette to what you usually use.

• You might want to go around your home seeking out objects in a colour you are drawn to and arrange them on your altar space.

• Experiment with a flashy red lip, an emerald jacket or a colourful throw upon your bed.

 # Journal Prompts

• What colours make up the palette of your home and wardrobe? What meaning do they hold for you?

• Has pregnancy changed the colours you are drawn to?

• What emotional experiences have I had this recently, how are they drawing my attention or teaching me?

• Who or what is activating more extreme reactions in me lately? What message might this hold?

• Am I honouring my internal messages, or am I finding ways to ignore, repress and discard them? How might I be more aware of their importance...

 Affirmation: *I welcome deeper connection and honour the messages this brings.*

Week 32
Becoming a Mother, Becoming Yourself

One of the greatest gifts of motherhood for me has been the fact that it has allowed me to become more fully myself. After my first child was born, I recognised that I am in control of what our days look like. I am the one leading the show. I am the one big enough and bad enough to have grown and birthed a human. Motherhood allowed me to settle into my skin fully, as if for the first time in a very long time (maybe for the first time ever). Having children was a homecoming, a reckoning with truth, and being responsible for young souls has become a beautiful and unexpected reclamation of self.

The things we lose to parenthood are often things we are done with anyway (some permanently, others temporarily). Change is an inevitable part of life and as parts of our existence drop away, we are left with a blank page. This page need not be a loss, nor is it emptiness. It is space to be filled. Some of this, in the start, becomes consumed with unenviable tasks such as bum cleaning, but that shifts, and we find a new stride to life. It is on the pages of parenthood that we can start to write our own stories anew.

As we become ourselves, we can parent how we wish, and grow into our own adulthood in playful ways. As a parent we get to re-live our childhood and reclaim parts of it that perhaps we wished had been different. It's a beautiful canvas upon which to paint, and as the adults we hold the brush. The growth that parenthood allows on our characters and wellbeing is immense and something to be treasured.

As you head towards the newest addition to your family, I recommend you do so with contemplation of who you really want to be. Whilst birth and early baby years may leave you feeling bedraggled, they are also moments of your life when formation is occurring. Life isn't supposed to be neat and easy, but it is a cauldron of possibility. In all my life, the greatest most life-changing event, the one that brought me into closeness with my truest self, has been parenting. Hands down. Nothing touches it, so I put last week's existential crisis aside a moment and recognise that *this* is always precisely where I need to be.

Overlooked by society and rendered as a domestic chore, motherhood is a place of transformation and great power. This may be the defining moment when *you* make sense, and life as you knew it shuffles to the side to be replaced with a more visceral and honest account of selfhood. Do not underestimate the value of the road ahead, even and especially the tougher parts of it, for you are a diamond being pressed into being. As time moves through you into one, two years, the gift you are given is one of freedom to finally become.

Meditation: *Seeing Yourself as Mother*

There are so many parts of yourself you have yet to meet. With every event, birth and year that passes you meet new versions of your truth. This meditation welcomes a new part of yourself, making space for growth and your own personal evolution.

Slip into your comfortable space, take a breath, and open your heart. Literally envision your heart opening as if it has a door or windows, release any dusty old energy, and open wide to the new.

Allow an image of you as mother to emerge in your mind's eye. Holding and guiding your child. Let yourself begin to feel this reality solidify. See the circles of love and support that you have around yourself: friends, family, professionals, all encircled with the love and support of the universe.

Sit in this circle of support, and when you feel complete, take a deep breath and be with your returned power as you return to everyday life.

Soulful Practice:
Who have I Been...
Who am I Becoming?

Take this week to reflect on who you have been and how you got to where you are. Looking back over life can provide some interesting insight. Especially as this relates to the funny little coincidences and synchronicities that have prodded and poked you into the space you find yourself in.

How have you grown? What came into your life, and what left? Who did you meet along the way? What were the most formative and exceptional happenings on your journey to motherhood? When you review this strange concoction of life happenings how do you feel? How might this same magic follow you onwards into the future? Write, journal, think and chat to like-minded friends about this fascinating topic!

 ## Creative Practice: *Me as Mother*

Take some time to think about the vision of motherhood that you are wanting to embody. Consider the mothers and mother ideals that you admire.

Create a vision board with images of mothers, yourself with children, things you would like to do with your children, quotations about motherhood that inspire you, values that you intend to live out, things that you want to share with your child. You might want to include images of, or quotes from, mothers you know or celebrity mothers who inspire you.

Gather glue, scissors, papers and magazines and a large sheet of paper and get busy cutting and sticking. Design this board as a direct reflection of your inner mother-self that is emerging. Allow it to reverberate your bountiful energy and longings back to you every time you witness it. This would make a very special backdrop to your altar.

 ## Journal Prompts

- What do I think a mother should/shouldn't be/do/look like?

- How has my own mother influenced my view of motherhood? What of her mothering do I want to emulate or avoid?

- Who are my positive maternal role models?

 Affirmation: *I am becoming the mother that I and my child most need me to be.*

Week 33
Overcoming Overwhelm

I was awake from 5am this morning because I was dreaming anxiously that my unborn child did not have enough hobbies! Similarly, my husband, who has exhausted himself trying to get the house ready for baby, spent yesterday in a state of overwhelm because the bedroom has not been decorated appropriately. At this stage in pregnancy, there seems to be a never-ending list of things to prepare for or get stressed about – real and imagined – and all the time and energy in the world to commit to worrying about it all.

Despite being a seasoned parent of two much loved children, with my own soulful and creative support systems, I am not above the occasional existential angst. I find these days and moments descend on me when I'm tired or triggered by some difficult event. This year has been peppered with such happenings. The past 24 hours have seen me lurching around in the 'what the heck is the meaning of my life' territory and coming up with very few concrete answers!

As you head towards the inevitable birth of your child, despite the joy and expectation you may hold, there is no shame in the recognition that life is about to change dramatically. I have spent the last decade building a writing career, and since finding out I am pregnant at forty-four, I find myself sat on the precipice of deep longing for my babe and the shift of gears this enables, besides a real fear that all my work was for naught. Am I here to create, or am I here to mother? Or maybe it's all just a freak accident that is none of my business and not that important anyway…

Whatever your space and place is in the world, it is about to change. If you have children already, this will shift too. The dynamics of all things take a boot to the backside when a baby arrives. Sitting and waiting for this can feel intimidating and so our brains go into overdrive worrying, fretting and planning.

We know, objectively, that this change in life may be exactly what is needed and yet the freaked-out human in us who is tired, stressed or hungry can manage to whip that lovely expectation into a frenzy from time to time. It's not really my intention to change your mood here or to shift you away from panic. Rather, I want to hold this part of the journey as normal and natural. I hope to create a small space where you can feel seen and held. Any doubt or fear you feel during this process of becoming is warranted, it is human, and I can only assure you, it won't last forever.

 # Meditation: *Calling in Strength*

As we sit on the edge of the unknown, overwhelmed with the enormity of what lies ahead and what is yet to be done before baby arrives, we can engage this meditation to help focus us on the power and solidity within...

I am especially inspired in creating this meditation by the Strength tarot card, traditionally shown as a character in peaceful calm white clothing, holding the jaws of a raging lion. This archetype and her story are an interesting one to delve into as we move into this meditation. How is our strength innate? How are we both the calm and the lion, sometimes at the same time? What might we do to soothe ourselves and temper the extremes of our reactions, whilst honouring any difficulties, fear or rage that live within? Think on the contradictions of your own emotions currently. What part of you is calm, rational and holding it all together? How are other parts spiralling into more difficult and negative feeling? Perhaps, as you move into this meditation, hold space for all those parts, none being wrong or right, but parts of your internal house, your personal make up, vying for attention, healing and witnessing. Strength cannot exist without some friction, and so it is in these moments of difficulty that courage, power and personal ability to overcome are conjured.

Sit with your back solid against a chair, tree or some other resting place. Take several deep breaths and bring yourself into this visualisation.

Imagine you are in a forest of dark sacred old trees and roots. It is tangled with connection and a profound sense of wisdom. Despite the interlaced branches and roots, the depths and darkness, the place feels, smells and is divine, ancient and full of peace. This forest knows itself and knows its power. It is reminiscent of something within you, some old and otherworldly presence of solidity.

Seek out your tree, the one that is your primordial wisdom keeper. Let yourself be guided to it. When you find your tree, move towards it, settling down amongst its roots. Feel yourself pulled into its energy field. Trust that the tree is holding you and bringing its wisdom through you via an immense and mighty connection. Notice the feel of the bark, the lichen and mosses on the floor, look up to see light cracking through the branches overhead, be at peace.

You may almost feel yourself melding into the trunk, becoming at one with this giant. The tree offers love and protection, the closer you sink into its aura, the more settled and grounded you feel. The opposing parts of you finding warmth and acceptance here, these parts striking an agreement to co-exist and in their contradictions, finding if not full peace, then so much strength.

Know that this tree is your source of strength. That even when you are not in togetherness, it abides within your consciousness, helping to source courage, bold choices and personal strength. Let the tree share with you its messages. These may come through as words, images or simply feelings. Feel the interaction, as at the same time you may offer thanks and love. You might also present the tree with any questions or worries you have at this time and trust that answers will find you. Spend as much time in the dark mysterious magic of your tree as you wish. Be with all your hopes and queries. Let your heart settle and feel held.

When the connection starts to wane, return to your body and in time, your day.

 ## Soulful Practice: *Engage*

Any overwhelm can be calmed and soothed by connection and engagement with what is real, solid and in front of you right now. Here are some ideas to get out of your head and unite back in with inner strength and continuity.

- Take three deep breaths. Put one hand on your heart, one hand on your womb and feel the ground beneath your feet.

- A sensory nature walk. Touch, feel and smell your way around a local beauty spot. Reconnect with the grounding energy of petals, leaves, ice or rain as you bring yourself back to harmony with a more level mood.

- Snuggle: snuggle physically with pets, partners, children or any other willing partner, including your old or future baby's teddy bears.

- Head back to bed and please yourself: close your eyes and dream, open them and daydream. Let the mood and moment shift without any effort on your part.

Creative Practice:
Create About How You Feel

That is what I did here in this week's section, and it helped. This whole book is testament to being creative with our feelings and happenings as the focal point. It really works to express ourselves and our moods through art, baking, growing, song or writing, and it is a soothing way to move those feelings on.

So, during your next period of overwhelm, step out of the whirl and use the junk in your head and heart to perform your creative magic. Write it, sing it and paint it out of you. Even if the mood does not shift immediately, you may find it opens doors to new parts of the conversation. You start to recognise that how you feel right now, is not alone in the potential feelings you could indulge. Interesting roads and directions may appear and the sense of overwhelm, panic, impending doom, when created outwardly, can become something more than it started as.

Journal Prompts

- I am most overwhelmed about…

- These things soothe me…

- What support can I reach out for?

- What can I put to one side for now?

- How is the shift into parenthood of this child exactly what I need right now?

 Affirmation: *I trust the deep unknown to*
gift me purpose and meaning.

Week 34
Baby Blessing

At 34 weeks your baby is making themselves known more than ever with their physical presence. It poses the question as to whether the soul has made an appearance yet? Some cultures believe the soul turns up months after the birth, whilst others argue it is around or after the six-month mark of pregnancy.

I have to say that with my children so far, I have felt the soul of each one, usually way before their conception. Whether this soul energy was embodied within the foetus, I couldn't say. Maybe it is suspended in the air around me or through some divine portal I couldn't possibly be sure about. All I know is that I kind of, sort of, knew them before they were even conceived.

I would argue that at least two of my children were hanging around for years as ideas and echoes of themselves. Whilst another came in for a shorter time just before conception but turned up so full of love and old soul magic. Once when this child was about two and I was having a close cuddly moment with her, she informed me that she used to do the same for me when she was my mother. So very matter of fact, so completely disarming. I loved it, I would love for her to have been my mother in some long-gone lifetime. Perhaps her soul is of a different ilk to the other two, who clamoured for my attention whilst waiting to be conceived, she calmly did not, but brings a certainty and roundedness that feels almost elemental.

It is my belief that whether that baby's soul is in the body, or elsewhere, the baby's soul is not negotiable, it is a soul that you have agreed or has been chosen in some way to show up eventually in your womb! They all feel and extend themselves differently, though this discussion is unlikely to have been had at your local parenting classes! If you have felt an inkling of the person you are birthing presenting their energy, gifting you snippets of visions of future possibilities, choose to believe it.

Whether you feel it important to connect and celebrate the physicality of the baby, or the spirit of them arriving, now is a great time to start to do so. I have thus far celebrated two deeply moving baby blessings with my babies. Though this time round I'm thinking of just going into full baby shower mode, I will probably combine aspects of both and conjure some between space, that is as sacred as it is a big fat party. Both types of baby celebration, a more spiritual blessing for baby and mother, or a full-on baby shower with gifts and games, can dig into the soulful and the creative practices this week, whilst the meditation may be a good one to do at the event itself, or at some private ceremony with very close family or friends.

 # Meditation: *Welcoming Baby In*

This short meditation may be used alone, or perhaps with a group of expectant mothers and/or family and friends who will be in the baby's life. If you have a baby and mother blessing style ceremony, then this could be adapted to be an opening ceremony. I wrote this for this book and then undertook it at my own baby's blessing, accompanied by shrieking, laughing children in the room next door, the television in the background and the meditation music taking a strange step towards rave halfway through! It was perfect. You may wish to encourage people new to meditation to take it lightly, to listen gently and not worry about 'getting it right'. Being in community and letting it be what it becomes is a beautiful surrender.

In a space of togetherness, lie or be seated in a circle. You may wish to have a person allocated to welcoming everyone to the circle, using words much like those scripted below. Have some gentle music playing in the background, incense burning and a candle for everyone to light at the end of the meditation. Briefly hold hands and breathe three deep breaths together.

"Welcome to the circle, we are taking a few moments in community to welcome this baby and their unique spirit into our lives and this world. We honour (your name) at this time and gather as she moves with baby into the next part of their journey together."

Everyone closes their eyes and brings themselves to the moment.

If possible, the same individual might lead with the following prompts.

"Place your hands on your hearts or wombs and take a few moments to envisage your part in welcoming baby. Think and feel in your own mind and heart about your gentle easy connection and friendship with baby and their parent/s. How might you offer love, support and community, here and further beyond this space into your other loving connections? Take a few silent breaths and be with this moment of potential and community."

Allow the group (or yourself if working individually) to dive deeply into personal private visions, hopes and prayers for mother and baby.

A minute or two later.

"We now take a moment to inwardly welcome baby and honour these sacred weeks before birth. You may wish to spiral inwards for a moment, bring yourself to your own imagined experience of being in the womb, and offer your own baby self a few words of wisdom. Let yourself voyage to an inner place of love that recognises the journey from womb to infant, to adult and around and around again. Allow any wisdom or insight to bubble through you. Be with this for a few breaths."

A minute or two later:

"Breathe into your own life experience and promise to honour what has arisen in guidance, love and respect to this baby and to all children, including your own inner child and that of the other adults you know and love."

Take a deep refreshing breath. Return to the room.

Candles to be passed around quietly.

Everyone to light their candle and to one at a time share a few words of love with the mother and personal reflection as they feel comfortable to do so...

 ## Soulful Practice: *Blessing*

Blessing is a tradition shared by all spiritual backgrounds. In many modern circles we have baby showers – marking the baby's imminent arrival, time to celebrate the mother, showering her with gifts and love in the run up to her birth.

I have now had three baby blessings for both my daughters and enjoyed undertaking some very special rituals and moments. You can find my first Baby Blessing recorded for a TV show called *She's Having A Baby – Episode Two*! Search on YouTube to see a much younger version of myself with my first child.

Much like a baby shower, people gather in honour of the birthing mother and baby. Gifts can be brought if wished, but this is not a necessity in any way. At each gathering to honour baby and myself, I requested that everybody bring a bead, and a little poem or passage to read.

The beads are strung together to represent qualities we wish for our baby and birth, and love of the collective. This can be kept for the baby, but also brought to the birth to connect to the energies of loved ones and garner strength.

The readings are for the baby and can be collected into a folder for their perusal one day. If people are comfortable, it is very emotional to hear people read theirs out.

I also arranged for everyone to receive a small candle to take home. The idea here is that when you go into labour then those with the candles are informed and they can light them. This helps to honour and bring in baby in a spiritual way, whilst holding the mother and her efforts close to heart. This is not essential, but a lovely option if you are open to it.

At my second daughter's blessing event we made flower crowns and my mother's civil partner arranged the most beautiful altar full of flowers, candles and power items. Some of the attendees also washed my feet, which was in service to myself as birthing mother.

There are so many ways to play with a baby blessing and make it special for you. The idea is that is far more ritualistic and spiritual than a baby shower. At the end of the ritual, like with any good party, there is food and cake and, if you like, you can ask everyone to bring a dish to share, to infuse the community aspect into the dining. Whilst mine were specifically more spiritual, I believe you can bring elements of these into sacred solo work, or to a bigger platform such as a party or otherwise.

 ## Creative Practice: *Group Creation*

As you entertain the possibility of a baby shower or blessing ceremony, you may like to consider how a part of this might include a creative activity that your friends and family can be involved with. Here are some ideas:

- **Messages to baby.** It may be something as simple as providing a journal or large sheet of paper and allowing people to write their own heartfelt messages and doodles upon it. Maybe you provide paint and let little ones run riot over it with handprints and footprints, welcoming in the newbie.

- **Bump painting.** Source some non-toxic body paints or henna and go wild. You may wish to decorate your own bump or allow others to make their marks. Make yourself the canvas and enjoy the very temporary artwork that you are! Be sure to get a photo of it to treasure.

- **Flower Pressing.** If anyone brings flowers, press them between the pages of an old book, and when dried, create an image for the baby's nursery or baby journal. Or arrange for a walk in nature with loved ones who will be involved in baby's life. Collect some seasonal leaves and flowers that catch people's eyes. Remember who chose what flower or leaf so that you can perhaps provide annotation for your child to contemplate in the future.

- **Baby Hat Messages.** A great idea instigated at my latest Baby Blessing by my mum's civil partner, was the purchase of snow white hats and some marker pens. Attendees then write messages on the hats for baby to wear or have as a keepsake in the future!

- **Face painting and fake tattoos.** Both my daughters were kept busy at this latest Baby Blessing, one performing facepaint on many of the other children and guests, whilst the other gave out pretty floral tattoos to the kids and adults alike.

- **Create an altar** filled with candles, incense and tarot/oracle cards, instruct people to help themselves to the cards and allow them to explore the messages that come up!

 # Journal Prompts

- How might I share my creativity and spiritual belief with loved ones during this time?

- What blessings will my baby's birth bring to my life/my family/my community?

- How might I offer love and support to other families and parents of young children in my circles?

- My words of welcome for baby would be...

 Affirmation: *I welcome community that honours, loves and supports this journey.*

Week 35
Planning Your Birth

Birth is the portal through which your baby comes into the world, as at the same time, you become their mother or parent. Birth has become highly medicalised and sanitised over the last century, and yet remains for many people experiencing it a hugely transformative and often spiritual act no matter what form it takes.

So let's begin this week by recognising that no birth is wrong, no birth is a cheat or 'less than' in spiritual terms. Too much pressure is placed upon the altar of the perfect birth, with women feeling guilty after their birth because they did not achieve whichever expectation they held for themselves. Often the perception is that a natural birth is the kingpin of all birthing (ideally accompanied by singing, breathing or orgasm-ing the baby out), and anything that interferes with this is perceived as less spiritual, less real, less pure. This continues the longstanding mythology that women must be perfect/always smiling/submissive, even in pain, even when potentially in danger. I'd like to scoot that from the building and declare that all births are spiritual, all birthing people are divine and the way in which you choose or end up giving birth is equal to anybody else's.

Birth is a voyage, and it can bring smooth seas or choppy waters. To a very real extent, you might predict the weather, but the reality of sailing that weather is unknown. There should be no comparison here, no high ideals. Birth is birth and you will do with it the very best you can. It will challenge you and conjure you to your depths of being, no matter what happens. Whatever route you take, or changes that occur, are all part of that incredible initiation. So please, go easy on yourself, the plans made this week are shiftable, as I believe they should be.

You may have given birth before, or this could be your first time. Nothing I can say will prepare you for what happens at each unique birth, but I do want to offer an alternative perspective. Birth is a sacred quest, a moment of deep unknowable wildness, no matter how it plays out – natural, caesarean, intervention laden or induced – it is an opportunity to seek deep faith within, to embody that faith and to birth your baby and rebirth yourself with fervent, feverish intensity.

It is important that you claim your power and your space within this most profound and soulful of events. This is your first great act of the journey moving forward: allowing your voice to be heard in advocacy for yourself, your child and the way in which you both are born.

As I write this, I am navigating a baby who alternates between being in a breech (upside down) and transverse (sideways) position. Whilst there are a few weeks ahead, this scenario is causing my ability to plan the birth I'd like to be uncertain and confused. A natural birth in breech position at the age of forty-four is far from ideal, and so I find myself doing what I can to induce the baby to move. I have engaged the help of magical friends, using oils (peppermint on top of bump, myrrh on the bottom) to help encourage a natural spin. I sit on a birth ball often and have sourced moxibustion sticks from my acupuncturist pal (smokeless mugwort loaded sticks used in Chinese medicine) to burn with her guidance in a particular position that will also help baby turn (consult your local recommended acupuncturist). I am also spending an inordinate amount of time with my bum in the air in accordance with the Spinning Babies website. I am doing what I can. What happens beyond this is something to accept and honour. The birth that I would like lies on the other side of whatever happens next, I am claiming my power, whilst equally releasing to a momentum that may not be mine to decide...

This week we will explore the ways in which you can begin to create and journey towards your birthing desires. Whilst the act of birth itself may take you down alternative routes than you plan for, there are ways in which you can hold space, conjure the ideal environment, and be heard and seen within the process as it unfolds.

Meditation:
Becoming One with Your Body

Your body is key to birth. It holds the answers and will not be forced or coerced into whatever your mind thinks is right. When birthing occurs, there is a very real call to let the body lead. Empowering your body is sometimes about making plans, other times, about advocating for yourself to doctors and midwives, and at other moments, it is simply about giving your body permission to be in charge, to do its thing. This meditation allows for the drop away from your head and into the wisdom and ferocious knowing of your physical instincts.

Take a moment to close your eyes and come to a centred place. Allow the energies of your mind to silence and drop inward. Feel into your physical self. Can you feel the baby kicking? Does anywhere ache? Which areas of your body feel good and contented? Be with any sensation that arises and breathe into it.

Explore your body physically with your hands, stroking your arms, legs, stomach, breasts, hips and face. Caress your physical entity that has carried you so very far in life. Feel out areas of tension and gently massage them. Keep your eyes closed and allow the moment to be meditative and one built upon sensation. Feel into yourself. Feel into the inner realms of your body – your womb, your heart, your guts, your muscles – is all well? Is anything trying to get your attention?

Run your fingers through your hair, over your feet or down your sides, look for points of stimulation that feel good, that help you feel calm or centred. Finding areas that feel thrilling or pleasant to the touch is a reminder that the body is here to be lived.

As you move over your bumps and curves repeat the following.

"I love you, I trust you, I thank you."

Sink into community and collaboration with your skin your bones and your muscle. Create connection with the wondrous vessel you inhabit that has been charged with such a beautiful task. Continue stroking and gently massaging yourself for as long as this feels powerful.

To close the meditation take a breath and hug yourself tight. Breathe in your own smell. Rock gently to and fro to bring yourself back to your space.

Repeat this daily for the week, perhaps in brief increments. Taking note of how you feel each time and any power spots that might be useful during birth to soothe or create courage. Allow these to be shared with a birthing partner, so that they might take over stroking, holding and massaging duties at your request during birth.

Soulful Practice:
Simple Ways to Reconnect to Your Physical Self

State of mind is a funny thing. We can become overly mired in certain ways of thinking, and whilst some of this needs to be undone by therapy or big self-seeking work, there are some simple ways to reconnect to the body, move out of fear and settle difficult feelings. Here I suggest some accessible practices you can undertake as you move towards birth that help you to ground and centre yourself back into the moment.

- Three long deep breaths in through the nose, out through the mouth. So simple, so accessible and it can be done anywhere. Taken in consciously, these breaths can whip a frenzied mood into something more ease-filled very quickly. Try it and see.

- Connect to the earth. Earth is our mother, our sustained and resource-filled home. Taking time to 'be' with her is powerful. You can conjure this through imagination, closing your eyes and spending a moment in an imaginary natural space. If possible, get outside and walk barefoot.

- Drink a large glass of water. Simplicity indeed. Many a headache, foul mood or uncertainty of feeling can be cured by hydrating!

- Consider whether you are tired or hungry. Easy to ignore, the symptoms of everyday needs can make our moods spiral profoundly. Serve your symptoms with much needed rest and nourishing food.

- Fiddle with a lovely crystal palm stone as an anchoring presence in your pocket or between your hands. I happily found a gorgeous labradorite palm stone on a dog walk recently, the dog insisted on sniffing at it over and over till I noticed and picked it up. It hasn't gone far from my pocket, and I love flipping it over in my hand, such a soothing and simple slice of adult style 'fidget toy'. Of course any pebble or rock will suffice, perhaps look out for the perfect one next time you are out walking.

Creative Practice:
Writing Your Birth Plan

Now is a good time to start pulling together a gentle guide to what you would like to happen and be attended to during your birth. Here are some possibilities:

- Consider where you intend to birth: at home, birth centre or hospital. Bring the place to mind regularly and imagine yourself there, safe, calm and supported.

- What is there…and what will you need to bring? Make a list of necessities should a hospital stay be required: spare clothes, pyjamas, underwear, a phone charger, headphones, large sanitary towels, diapers, baby clothes, a wash bag etc.

- Think about the person or people you choose to attend, and what will happen with pets and existing children.

- You may have hopes towards a water birth, or the ability to move around and shift position. Put these ideas and desires on your plan.

- You may wish to have a plan to discuss or delay medical procedures, or have ideas in place around their happening, should you and the doctors and midwives recognise they are necessary. You might like to consider how you will counter any request to change your plans and take on board any arising news or complications.

- You may also include self-care items to help support you and keep you centred and calm: desires for lighting, oils, soothing balms, birthing meditations or guidance, birthing ball or stool, the music you want played, the ice chips or drinks you will need and the company you keep.

All of this can be accumulated into a birth plan, and shared with those who support you. Keep it to hand and research ideas and items you could add or change upon it. Note which parts are definitive and which parts flexible. Make this plan a living entity. Discuss this with your support team, midwives, doula and maybe a few other people who have given birth and might have some interesting ideas of their own. Collate the ways you can prepare for all birthing circumstances.

Create a collage of ideas and hopes, mantras and words of affirmation to keep close to hand when the time comes.

 # Journal Prompts

- Have you birthed before? If yes, how was it and how do you feel about this next time? If no, what are your expectations and hopes?

- What anxieties do you feel towards birth?

- Who might you connect or speak with to talk things through?

- Is there a particular aspect of birth you are looking forward to as a unique experience?

 Affirmation: *I am free to find power in my birth experience.*

Week 36
Nesting

The time when you meet your baby is just around the corner, there are only a few weeks left of pregnancy and now is the time to make some practical shifts in your home. I appreciate you may have already been busy with variations of this, perhaps painting a nursery or stocking up on diapers and other essentials. This week we will bring our energy to the concept of 'nesting'.

Aside from the material everyday, it is important that we create a nest that feels feathered, not just by blankets and softness, but love, support, soulful belief and creativity. It is important that you feel held within this space just as much as your child, and that everyone living in your home has some sense of continuity amongst whatever the change of circumstances brings.

This week we contemplate the big shift that is coming and find ways to prepare and explore that change in beautiful empowering ways. As you live through this week, I would guide you to think deeply about the type of home you want to raise a child in. What needs to change in your immediate vicinity, perhaps even internally, to allow a collaborative growth from everyone involved? This may involve tricky conversations and some promises of deep continued healing. It is wiser to have these conversations now, than to wait five years and be tripped up by toxic old ways you had turned a blind eye to.

This does not mean that you need to change overnight, or that your home must be rebuilt in the next few weeks. Rather the nest you are aiming to make is one of continual growth and aspirations of becoming better than you were before. No family or parent is perfect, yet parenthood subjects us to a deep need to change, where we resist, we create difficulty and sometimes pain. Being open to the softness of becoming better, becoming different, is a good place to start, a great place for baby to land.

Spend some time this month considering the home you currently have, in all its energies, timekeeping, attitudes and habits. What goes on beneath your roof that is gorgeous and profound, and what is perhaps a little more unkempt and trickier?

Is there peace, or are there areas of divisiveness that might be ironed out, or at least spoken about and resolved to healing? Is this something you can deal with alone or with a partner, or is a call for support from others necessary? Move into these choices without judgment, recognising that this is the work of parenthood, to find peace, to become more filled with truth and a knowledge of what is and is not appropriate.

How is your home sweet home conducive to the barnstorming arrival of an innocent infant? What might need to be shifted or compromised? Just as you seek to use non-toxic materials for the baby's nursery, and block power sockets from curious little fingers, how might you protect your child from toxic emotion or dangerous behaviours? What parts of your inner story may need to become more flexible and to shift and change? And on the fun side, how can you make perfect little last tweaks to the space around you to most boldly and beautifully welcome your new soul?

 ## Meditation: *Fill Your Home With Light*

This meditation is designed to bring light to your home, through setting your internal expectation of the home as a light-filled place of magic and miracle. Before settling down, you may wish to burn a candle, and in doing so honour the love with which you will always make effort to bring to your space.

Closing your eyes, and relaxing, bringing your body to full rest. Take a few deep breaths.

When you are ready, envision yourself in your home, as you are, feeling empowered and strong. Take a moment to verbally or mentally call in healing energies:

"I call in divine light to my home, my body and the individuals who live here. May these spaces be filled with love, inspiration and so much safety."

Visualise the light coming from a divine source, be that god, the heavens or the cosmos. Imagine the light touching and swelling into every room. Trusting that it leaves no cupboard or surface untouched. This light helps to seek out residual negative energy and remove it, whilst aligning the walls, floors, and air with clean, clear energy. Allow the light to flood in, to swirl around you and within you, trusting it to harm none, but to bring appropriate changes and alignment.

Take a moment to set your own personal expectations for your home within your own heart and mind, find the areas of peace that are non-negotiable, and let them infiltrate your consciousness. Pray these expectations into your spaces and let them infuse all that they touch.

Sit with this until such time as it feels complete. Consider your home sanctified. Imagine the light diffusing away, taking with it any toxicity. Bring yourself back to the moment with a refreshing breath.

Soulful Practice:
Blessing Your Home
(and all who dwell there)

This week I propose ideas that you can undertake to make your house feel more habitable on an energetic level.

- **Incense.** I love incense, I burn it nearly every day and find it sets intentions and hopes very well. It helps you feel aligned to your core principles, whilst also giving the home a fragrant lift that has spiritual undertones.

- **Smudging.** You might also enjoy the idea of using a ceremonial tool such as ethically sourced Palo Santo or sage to 'smudge' the energies in your home. These natural products are believed to remove stagnant energy, and even difficult and stubborn spiritual energies that have attached to your space. Waft them through each room, over your body and open the window and doors to fully allow the release of any toxic build ups.

- **Essential Oils.** I adore using essential oils. You can add these to a diffuser or add to a very basic water solution that you use to clean surfaces, floors and doors with. You can research the blends or individual oils that would welcome the vibrations you are seeking for. I personally enjoy the simplicity of lavender, rosemary, frankincense, rose and cinnamon, though there are many oils that might meet your preferences and become powerful allies when used and mixed by you.

- **Air.** Purposefully open all the windows and doors to shift energy, and aid the removal of anything negative and toxic (best done alongside using your smudge stick).

- **Fire.** Burn candles in all rooms with a view to burning off old unhelpful energies.

- **Sound.** Another wonderful way to move energies is with sound. You may wish to sing your way around your home, bang a drum or a saucepan with a wooden spoon, or play some affirming soundtrack whilst you gently dance your way around your rooms.

- **Feng Shui.** Teach yourself the art of peaceful space habitation using a book or online Feng Shui resources. Shift furniture and ornaments (carefully and with help if necessary) to create a greater flow of energy and alignment in your space.

- **Nature.** Add some living plants to your rooms to help freshen the air and create life in dead spaces.

- **Mantra.** Work with a mantra as you move through any of the above practices. I occasionally combine several of them and walk round muttering something that feels powerful and relevant. Invent your own, or use something such as this…

"My home is a place of safety, love and power. Only those with good intentions cross the threshold."

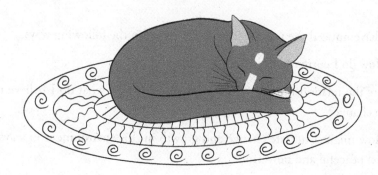

 # Creative Practice: *A Love Contract*

First and foremost, the home should be a place of sanctuary and protection from the outside world. This week's Creative Practice is to make it so by clearly setting your vision and boundaries for your home.

You could draw up a contract with yourself, and any other person who abides with you. The aim of this is to hone in on what you expect from your sacred space. Within this work you can consider what each individual needs and requires from their home, but also you might set expectations of love, behaviour and care-related goals on baby's behalf. Your contract could focus on the kinds of feelings you want to honour and evoke in your home, but also on those actions and behaviours that will not be tolerated.

Much of this often goes unsaid, with people holding invisible expectations of one another for decades. Allow this to be a living document, one that can be summarised in a few words, but drawn out for revisiting from time to time as new issues arise. This contract honours all the life forms in your space and becomes a safe working document with which to negotiate the importance of everybody's needs as you strive to live together peacefully.

You might want to draft a list of house rules or values – there are some lovely ones on the market that you can buy as well. Paint them or write them out in beautiful calligraphy and hang them on the wall to affirm the values you want to cultivate in your home.

 # Journal Prompts

- I have noticed the nesting instinct in myself in the following ways...

- How do I currently feel in my home?

- Are the relationships here in a good place? If not, what do I believe needs to change?

- How might I initiate change and growth in this environment in ways that feel peaceful and powerful?

- What values and qualities do I wish to cultivate in my home?

 Affirmation: *My home is a sacred, safe and loving space.*

Week 37

Love

Pregnancy has always been a lesson in love for me. In carrying and bearing a child, my heart opens to the innocence and innate precious nature of all things. Love is an energy that infiltrates more than just those 'special' relationships, it imbues our days with a thirst for connection and feeling that goes beyond the usual shallows. We are taught from a young age that love is to be reserved for only the special few: the perfect partner, our family, close friends and of course, our children. But I believe love is a mission of compassion and mystical coming together of connection, people and relationships. It need not be limited by anything whatsoever. The further we let love soak into our every interaction, the closer we come to our higher selves.

It is not just my child that I love and feel for, it is all children. It is not just human children I care about, it is the children of all living creatures, and the very fact that every living thing that exists was once a baby, a sapling, something small and vulnerable. The potential that sits within every footed and rooted life is beyond measure. Whatever comes of that potential is irrelevant. There is something to be loved about it all. This is quite the perspective to have, one that forgives, embodies compassion and grows from within.

This week we will explore beyond the shallows of love and find it within ourselves, as a resource of tremendous clarity and power. For as we move through pregnancy to meet with our child and welcome them into our world, we may feel real concern about how to love this being. There may be issues arising as to how we were loved or unloved as children. We may have no true understanding of what unconditional love is and then upon meeting be bowled over by intensity. If we have other children, we might worry about how our love for them could possibly be shared with another.

Our mission is to gently explore love as tidal force washing through our heart, mind, spirit and body, whilst being open to whatever that force of love chooses to bring with it. In this time, we welcome the possibility that our love is endless, and has no real limits. No matter the models of love we have received from family or partners, now is the time to forage into the wilderness of the untapped love within.

As you move through this week, allow love to be a state you keep returning to. Wear your love like water, let it flow in and around you, but trust your instinct to know not to be abused or taken advantage of. Rein your love, guard it, but feel it through all your bones and each singular moment. Allow the idea of endless love to alter and affect your choices, and practice trying to see the world through the eyes of a person not embattled or embittered, but via a looping harmony of love.

 # Meditation: *A Seed of Love*

Breathe deeply and close your eyes. Sit in peace until you feel calm, easy and ready to unfurl into this story...

Envision a small seed, a kernel of love within you. Remember that seedlings grow, they unfold and develop into something bigger and more impressive. You don't need to know what your seedling will become, but take time to imagine its gentle growth within you, planted somewhere in your midsection, your heart or solar plexus.

As you breathe, you bring energy to this seed of love. It starts to crack open, releasing boundaries that have previously held it in tight. The seed becomes a sapling, taking root in your body and growing into your cells, your structure, redefining everything there with love. Let this wild jungle of love bloom within, curling into your muscle and bone, your heart and your soul...

Breathe long deep breaths, allowing the wilderness within to blossom. Feel the lush and immense spiralling of love within as you surrender to the possibilities this will bring. Allow anything standing in the way of your plant's growth to be released, used as fuel and let go of. Feel yourself fresh and new in the raw, vulnerable and natural power of love blossoming from within.

When you are ready, bring your attention back to your body, hold yourself, pat yourself down, take a breath and return to the room.

Soulful Practice: *Check In*

Take time every morning to check in with yourself in the way you might expect a beloved to do. Review how you are and consider what you might do to lighten your load. Offer yourself love and consider yourself worthy of your own attentions, kindnesses and sympathy. Sweep yourself up in an embrace, make a self-hug part of your day, breathe yourself in and kiss your arms. It may feel silly, but there is something wonderfully soothing about gifting yourself this physical holding and affection. Make it a part of your daily routine this week.

Check in too with the ways in which you express your love currently. Are you particularly affectionate with your partner or your pet? Are there certain circumstances in which you feel uncomfortable expressing how you feel clearly? Or maybe love for you is expressed through desire, sex, making a meal, the simple act of kind words or hand holding. See how love works its way through you and explore the peculiarities of your own love style. Sit with expressions of love from others and pull that energy in to warm your loins and elevate you, in turn, sharing that outward, projected onward to those people and things which feel worthy.

Creative Practice: *Create with Love*

Undertake a creative interest that you love and do so with love. There is no point me directing you to something outside your comfort zone when there may be a pile of knitting or paint with your name on it. Think about what skill you'd enjoy practicing, or that thing you have been putting off doing, but that your heart is set upon.

This is what we do this week, create for the sheer fun, the beauty, the harmony it provokes within your inner world. Take your loving energy and unfurl it into something that you already enjoy doing. Perhaps create something that is upon a theme of love, or maybe just be swept by pure enjoyment into creating something, anything, be that cupcakes or clay vases, it doesn't matter. Let your love become a thing.

Journal Prompts

- When in my life have I experienced a huge and unfiltered love for all that is (even if just for a moment)?

- How do I currently withhold love, or use my love sparsely?

- If I were to love myself completely, how might all my interactions be felt differently?

- Have I ever experienced unconditional love myself and what has it taught me?

- In what ways am I led by love? At other times what is it that leads me?

 Affirmation: *I am led by love.*

Week 38
Trust the Unexpected

In the tarot there is a card called The Wheel of Fortune. This card, for me, speaks to the reality that no matter how we plan our lives, something else is usually likely to happen. There is divine happenstance within this card, though as humans we tend to only see the difficulty of life being interrupted or becoming outside of our control. Despite the fact that unexpected events occur frequently throughout our lives and may be divinely guided in some ways, we continue to see them as a nuisance or worse, a bombshell to our better laid plans.

The unexpected is a seriously real part of life, one we meet daily. Yet, perhaps due to our schooling and conditioning, we feel that we should be the ones in control. Sometimes, of course, we are! But once that control is wrestled from us, we shake our heads in disbelief, declare it all so unfair and psychologically wrangle with the gods to try to fix the situation.

I recently did just this. My elder daughter was on a big school trip for a week, the first of its kind, and a massive experience for us all. On the third day away, I had a call from the school saying she was vomiting. I tried to explain it away, it must be something, anything, other than a bug. I so wanted her to have this experience. Needless to say she continued to vomit and I dashed on a mercy mission to collect her. She was happy and relieved to see me and admittedly looked terribly sick. Yet for the rest of the day, I wrestled with the idea that she should be on the trip. This was fused awkwardly with the idea that she was much better off with me at home. My mind struggled to accept the unexpected turn of events, and despite evidence that this was what was happening, and what must happen, it took a little while for me to accept this unexpected scenario.

As life interrupts us, we may find ourselves looking to the past, trying to see where we went wrong, what we could or should have done to prevent the change in pathway. Inevitably we contemplate the ways in which we could get life back onto the track we had hoped it was on before things went awry. The more we try to intervene in what has happened, the more chaotic life conspires to be (and the less calm and settled we become).

This week our quest is to accept the unexpected, to trust it. Even to recognise that there is purpose within it. Whilst we may not know what that is, we will try not to fight arising influences, and instead witness them for what they are. What they are may be better plans, helpful redirections and forks in our understanding that inevitably take us out of what we 'think' and closer to what we 'feel'.

My experience with my daughter helped me to see that whilst I thought she should be on the trip having fun with her friends, the reality was she wasn't and couldn't be and that, when I really felt into it, the healthiest happiest place for her was at home. Just because we think a thing doesn't make it true, let's use this week to surrender to the flux and change that wants to meet us, let's welcome it and explore the new routes with intrigue.

As you may remember my baby has, at the time of writing, been breech for weeks and weeks, the stress of trying to turn him has felt quite substantial. The bigger picture presented here, I have discovered, is that baby will turn when, and if, baby wants to. No matter how many oils I apply, inversions I undertake or moxibustion sticks I burn, there is a factor of potential that is far outside my scope or ability to control. Today I headed for a final scan under offer of manual turning (ECV) should he still be breech. I had relented to the Wheel of Fortune and had ceased doing much to change or control this situation. The scan showed immediately he has turned to the correct head down position, he took the odds (which are low at 38 weeks) and he damn well did it!

Intriguingly, last night I dreamt I was riding an incredible black horse, fully in control of her movements and yet unaware and in awe of just 'how' I was mastering her. This is Wheel of Fortune energy, giving over to an unknown plan and finding ways to honour each moment as it takes place free from meddling, perceptions and plans. The Wheel of Fortune is all the surprises and unexpected magic that take us through important challenges and experiences, It is the dark horse of destiny that braids together what we did not want with what we really need. And so it is...

 ## Meditation: *The Wheel of Fortune*

The Wheel of Fortune allows us to experience forces that are beyond our own knowing or control. This may at times feel chaotic or difficult, and yet, the general rule of thumb is that when we let go of trying to be in control, life becomes easier. The flow we all wish for, the ease and the alignment, comes when we release the reins, when we let life be what it is, without our direction.

This week's meditation is a practice in letting go, with the aim of letting this practice stem out into our everyday.

Bring yourself to rest, close your eyes and take some breaths. Allow yourself to move into a state of calm. Know that you do not need to do anything or oversee anything right now. You simply are. Despite a moment of nothingness, life continues.

Envision yourself in a forest. As you meander through the trees, you notice a clearing. In this clearing you see a wheel. The wheel is spinning and upon it there are a hundred thousand possibilities. Wherever the wheel lands is beyond your control.

As you move towards the wheel some energy beckons you closer. You are connected to the wheel by long ribbons. You look down and see words written on each ribbon in spiralling script. You realise that these ribbons represent your expectations, and the matters in which you try to influence the wheel. As the wheel turns, your ribbons are getting tangled, confused and mixed. You understand that for clarity to resume you must trust the turn of the wheel and release your expectations. You must let go of control.

The wheel slows down, but you are still attached via the lengths of ribbons. In your mind's eye imagine possessing scissors, a sword or some other cutting device. Taking a deep breath, it is your time to chop and cut through your ribbons, entrusting the outcome and events of life to the wheel, to the gods and to the wisdom of inevitability. As you slice the ribbons you may wish to say or think the following words:

"I trust in an outcome bigger than my own perception and knowledge."

Feel the energy shift as you cut through the ribbons and allow destiny to take back control. You step off the wheel and acknowledge that giving over control to some higher power feels liberating. You may wish to watch the wheel turn for a while, free from your attempts at control. Honour this moment. Trusting that all will be as it is meant to be, irrespective of your choices, decisions or attempts to coerce or direct.

Sit with the words a moment longer. Yawn, stretch gently, return to your day.

 ## Soulful Practice: *Hand it Over*

With every perceived shift or interruption to your plans, make efforts to consciously hand the situation over to an unseen higher force. Witness your thoughts around change and hiccups to your plans and instead of entertaining frustration, be curious about what might happen next. Take note of this in a journal so that you might bring this process into full light. Observe your inner processes as frustration gives way to acceptance and an allowance of a different experience. Let yourself to be soft and flexible with what occurs.

 ## Creative Practice: *Automatic Writing*

Automatic writing is often used in spiritualist circles to receive psychic messages as well as in psychotherapy to access the subconscious. My suggestion is to practice some automatic writing this week to get in touch, not with the deceased, but with the alive parts of you; the more inner, intuitive parts that hold a higher wisdom than the ego led, purposeful driven aspects.

To perform your automatic writing, perhaps do so after a relaxing or meditative session, all you need to do is sit with a pen and paper, and close your eyes, perhaps have a question in mind. Allow words to flow through you to the paper, crystallising new understandings. Some of this may read like gobbledegook, other passages or sentences may hold great wisdom. Sit with the writing until it ceases to flow. Give it a little time. Trust that you are contacting a wiser inner part of you and see what she has to say!

 ## Journal Prompts

* How have I been resisting change? Have I ever tried to accept interruption and change, and how did this make matters easier?
* Do I bargain with the universe and what does this look like for me?
* Is there something right now that I could try to accept and trust?

 Affirmation: *I accept change and am curious about its higher purpose for me.*

Week 39
Curl into Self

Pregnancy can make you feel like public property. If people aren't being handsy with the bump, they are striking up conversations and telling you their experiences. This is no bad thing, but the pressure to listen, to smile, to be commented upon can in time become quite draining. You may also feel great anticipation at the arrival of your baby, whist dreading other aspects of the looming changes. The reality of pregnancy at this late stage is all things: love, fear, excitement, loss of control, gaining of connection, unwanted opinions, unexpected symptoms, tiredness...

You may feel quite fractured, as if your parts have been cracked and thrown all around the place, and even if that is not the case, you may wish to take action to reboot and avoid some later exhaustion. It may feel too that the worries and anxieties you are carrying are beyond help or assistance.

This third pregnancy has felt lonely as it ends. I am not without help or support, however, it's been a time of great inner tumult, bone numbing tiredness and intensive and hermetic inner experience. The bountiful offers of assistance I am surrounded by from friends and family have been unable to match the existential and, at times, overwhelming nature of impending birth. I have become allergic to kindness, advice or offers of support, whilst equally activated and frustrated by people's well-meaning presence and platitudes.

This, I am finding, is a moment I must walk entirely alone and in a way that others may not comprehend. So, whilst it has been solitary, I have in equal parts withdrawn myself from opinion and consumption. I have turned inward, reliant on self and created freedom to be strong, afraid, loving and brave all within a spiralling swirl of whatever it is I am becoming.

This week our practice and processes will focus on coming home to ourselves, being gentle with where we are, honouring the fear, honouring the changes, honouring the love, and regrouping inwardly to connect to the inner source that is driving our resilience and our baby's continued healthy passage to birth.

I have felt in this week, and moments surrounding it, that I simply want to curl up. I went to a sound bath and enjoyed an hour of just being in my own body, curled on my side like a spiral shell. It was such a basic, passive act but in many ways became a symbol of what I needed. I needed to make space for myself. To place boundaries around my shell, to call my energy back in and be with where I am emotionally, mentally, physically and of course, spiritually.

I invite you to settle a little at this point, to move inward, to curl up into yourself, much like how your baby is curled into you. This is all about reclaiming your energy, reserving it, and most importantly protecting it.

It is a power move to make space for oneself, to call all your parts back without requiring a third party to help, without needing anyone's permission. Navigating this terrain of love and fear, excitement and overwhelm will be entirely unique and changeable by the hour. Let this week be testament to your spiralling inward and starting to access your own capacity for wellbeing, rest and protection.

 # Meditation: *Spiralling*

This week our meditation helps us return to power, by actively calling in any parts of self that have been lost along the path of life.

Curl into a comfortable position and relax. Take three deep breaths and rest without any expectation.

Imagine yourself beginning to spiral inwards. You might envision your body lit up by light and energy, in all kinds of colours that suit your soul. These colours begin to spin gently and move deeply inward, finding a centre point within you, perhaps in your heart, womb or belly. Recognise that you always return to self. The aspects of you that have been harmed or that have been forgotten, dropped aside or released, always return back, to fill you with your own personal power.

The swirl of energies moving through you knows no boundaries, it can visit the past or even the future, creating a constant spin of return, all of yourself, becoming whole again. As you witness and feel this return to self, you can call your parts back in. Say this or something similar…

"I call back all my parts, all my power and all aspects of my true self."

Repeat this several times if you feel called to. Allow a new flow of energy to swirl and spiral within you. Enjoy the feeling of coming home, back to your body and your spirit. Allow the gentle return of all your energy, strength and possibility. Let this spin and cycle, and trust that your aspects of inner being will return in their own time over the coming weeks in alignment with your readiness to receive them.

Allow this to work through you until such time as it seems to ebb, then bring yourself gently back to the room with an energising breath.

 ## Soulful Practice: *Little Rituals*

There are rituals and moments of private spiritual practice that I have built up over time that I find affirming. Maybe you have some of your own? This week is a good time to visit these simple rituals and give yourself space and time to indulge them. Ritual allows us to feel connected to the creation and manifestation of our lives, in ways that equally offer the reins to a higher power. In ritual we can become clear about our desires and hand those desires out to the universe, trusting that what is returned is right. Ritual also allows a divine connection that helps us to feel less alone, a way to connect with our faith in tangible and practical ways. If this is new to you, here are some lovely ideas.

- Light incense, a candle or create an essential oil mix. Infuse your home and spirit with their energies, and do so with an intent to honour your spirit, to carve out time for yourself and feel reconnected with your magic.

- Play with oracle cards or tarot. Ask a few questions, and see what comes up. A good question may be: "What do I need to know right now to make the most of this time?" Or, "What am I not seeing about the power and potential of my current circumstances?" I enjoyed taking some nature based oracle cards to reflect the events of my birth (I was surprisingly nervous given it was my third). The arising cards were spiritual, and a reminder of my power and the eventual blessings birth leads to. Let this interaction be light and airy, take the information being presented as a reflection of what you already known to be true, and recognise what this mirror might be encouraging you to shift or grow in your life.

- Use a pendulum to source direct answers from the divine. I would recommend tying a piece of string to a ring you often wear or using a special pendant necklace. Ask the pendulum to move one direction for yes and another for no. Now is not the time to go too deep or dark. Only ask questions that will offer up responses you can work with in your current situation.

- Walk barefoot on grass and imagine any pain or difficulty seeping out of you through your feet, being returned to Mother Earth for healing and transmutation.

- Write a letter to the universe with your hopes and requests upon it, take it outside and safely burn it.

- You may also choose to write down something you hope to grow within your life and then plant it out like it were a seed, in your garden or at a local park.

Creative Practice: *A Walk*

This week we are taking the pressure off doing anything too external, as we cosset and reenergise the inner world. Taking a walk through a local park or beauty spot, whilst allowing yourself to really engage with the nature around you is food for the soul. Indeed, most of my creative ideas come to me doing just this. Allow yourself to be fermenting ideas and gestating them, rather than doing anything with those ideas. Walk, listen to your inner voices, put your phone away, and simply be with the moment, the birds, the grasses and the particularities of the season.

Journal Prompts

- How do I feel conflicted and fractured this week?

- What might I do to support myself and feel more whole?

- How am I distracting myself or not allowing myself to be fully present?

- Putting everything down and sitting in silence and stillness for two minutes: *I feel...*

 Affirmation: *I am my home,*
I am my power, all I need is here.

Week 40
On the Edge of Birth

This week you may be on the edge of birth (if it hasn't happened already!). Birth is not about control or creating any form of perfected version of life-bringing. This is a nonsense fed to us by a capitalist society intent on holding women to high standards. Should these standards not be reached, we are left to contemplate our failings, to feel guilt and shame. Let me say it again: birth is not about control. The opposite in fact: the most powerful birth is about wild surrender.

In birth we learn to become one with the pulse of the universe – expansion and contraction – moving in waves through our wombs and bodies. This need not apply just to natural birth but to the variations of birth our modern world offers. A caesarean section, birthing emergency or use of medicalised options still require that wild surrender, the courage to trust, and the handing over of oneself to a wisdom and power greater than anything we envisioned. We must surrender wildly to the rigours of our bodies, and other times to the situations we find ourselves in. The mastery we do have, no matter how birth occurs, is in entering a state of divine ferocity, a state of mama bear energy that is free from everyday constraints and takes us towards our child with a boost of 'I didn't know I had it in me' expansive energies.

This wild surrender asks us to give our bodies over to a process: a process that is innate, unpredictable, powerful, exhausting and ultimately joyous. Each birth, like each mother and baby, is unique.

The one-upmanship amongst new mothers, played into by those selling perfect birth packages, and an over-inquisitive media that likes birth to be sanitised, has no place between your legs or in your womb. There is no room for regret or worry or guilt as it relates to birth. Birth is an initiation, the likes of which only those doing the birthing will ever truly understand.

Birth is a depth diving transcendent experience, and nobody should dictate what that looks like. It can be the making of you, but only if you allow it to overcome you. Which means flowing with what is really happening, not with what you thought you'd like to happen or what others encourage. Birth is a portal, a powerhouse and a place of deep inner change, no matter how it occurs.

Moving towards birth with acceptance and an understanding of this power is vital. As you birth your baby, vaginally, with assistance or by caesarean section, you are giving yourself to the life-changing power of wild surrender. There is no wrong here. Birth is beyond words, expression, control or expectation. Give yourself to it as it meets you. From this place you too will be reborn.

 ## Meditation: *Elemental Birth*

Birth is beyond you, it is elemental. Use this meditation to welcome in the raw power of the elements, the very make up of your being so that they might support you as you allow life to be born through you. Sit upright or with cushions for support. This meditation is active, though you may close your eyes to connect to your body.

Call in the elements in the following way: "I call in and welcome the elements of life and nature to support me as I move towards birthing my child."

Take a moment to feel the energy of the elements gathering. Then work through them with the following script.

"I call in Water, the energy of fluidity and flow, I welcome Water's wisdom within my body as I prepare to birth."

In your mind's eye, breathe in the element of Water for a few moments allowing the energy to flood you and empower your whole self.

"I call in Earth, the energy of grounding, growth and deep support. I welcome Earth's wisdom within my body as I prepare to give birth."

Breathe in the element of Earth for a few minutes, allowing yourself to feel the ground beneath you and the solidity of your physicality.

"I call in Air, the energy of spirit, life and living animation. I welcome Air's wisdom within my body as I prepare to give birth."

Breathe in the element of Air for a few minutes, allowing it to energise you and lighten your sense of being.

"I call in Fire, the energy of creativity, purpose and change. I welcome Fire's wisdom within my body as I prepare to give birth."

Breathe into Fire for a few minutes allowing the energy to heighten you and develop your sense of elemental power.

Repeat as many times as necessary, attempt to memorise the aspects that are helpful for you to reference when you are in the birthing process.

Soulful Practice: *Call in Spiritual Guides, Advisors and Assistance*

As you sit on the precipice of birth now is a bountiful time to call in whatever spiritual help you wish. Surrender your worries and fears to guides, angels, ancestors or your highest self. You may wish to do this through prayer, or a ritual wherein you call in your helpers and ask for support. Light candles, breathe deeply, maybe pull a tarot or oracle card. Be open and honest and vulnerable with your unseen support team. Ask for whatever you need, be it strength, power, magic or simply a loving presence. Keep this conversation going whenever you feel it necessary. Surrender to spiritual support knowing that support will be given, and alongside this, knowing that your body will do the work. Allow your mind to step aside and let the wonder commence!

Creative Practice: *The Elements*

You might enjoy thinking about ways in which you can bring the elements into your birth preparation. Here are some ideas you can play with to have on hand during birthing. Think about which you like, or come up with your own ideas and then make a chart, list or collection of items that you can have ready when the time comes…get creative!

- **Air.** A cooling fan, an open window or door, the depth of your own breaths to help conjure strength and power.

- **Fire.** Candles to usher in baby, to make the moment feel cloistered and sacred. You may require this in the form of warmth, a hot water bottle or warming electric pad.

- **Earth.** Grounding physical support of your partner or a loved one. Someone to hold your hand or an item to grasp onto. Consider birthing positions that help you feel empowered and bring you into contact with the ground or surface beneath you.

- **Water.** Ice, fresh water to drink, cooling cloths or a water birth. Stepping into the shower to soothe if able. Rain sounds or watery sounds playing in the background to promote flow.

Journal Prompts

- What vision do I have for my birth?

- Have I ever experienced surrender before? How does surrender feel to me right now as I approach this birth?

- What is holding me back?

- How am I trying to control my circumstances and why do I think this makes a difference?

- What is my promise to myself at this pivotal time?

Affirmation: *Earth, Water, Fire and Air support me and my baby as we birth life together.*

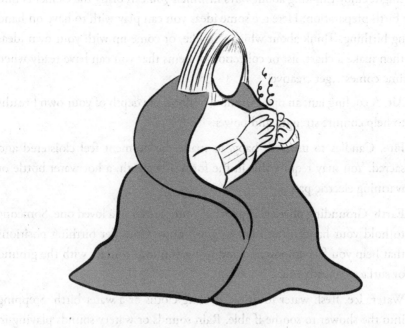

Weeks 41 & 42

Both my previous pregnancies have wandered into the post 40-week territory. My first child was over two weeks late, and I believe she may have chosen to stay longer had induction of labour not forced her out. My second daughter was a week past due date, and she found her way naturally just a few hours before she was due to be induced. When I look back on the 'overdue' period, I see it only as rose-tinted and sweetly gorgeous. A little extra time spent in a state of gestation, much like a flower that blooms longer than expected, this time allows for prolonged wonder…but can often be pressured from outside.

You may not feel the same way. This third pregnancy has me hoping for an earlier arrival, as this pregnancy is more physically taxing than I have experienced before. If previous births have taught me anything, it is that birth picks her own sweet time. Even induction is not a guarantee of a date – my first taking place very slowly over a week. Caesarean section may seem a guarantee of a birthday, yet even that can be trumped by a surprise natural labour. There are no certainties in this race to life.

As you move through these days or weeks that come after your baby's due date, let them be a meadow. Let the rolling expanse of time be something to delight in, rather than fight or clamour against. Let the reins fall far from your hands and trust that your baby will arrive, in their own style and timing, and the rest is for you to yield to. Give yourself over to the meadow of possibility and in this space observe the small, the inane and the holy moments that fly up like butterflies from the grass beneath your feet.

Walking through this moment of 'who knows' can feel all kinds of ways. For me it has at times been beautiful, a little more time with my babe in my belly has been a gift from the gods. Whilst in other moments, admittedly, it has been challenging, as sleep is compromised and my lungs are squashed beyond themselves. This time, however, is finite. Your baby is coming soon, so allow yourself to bring all your creativity to nesting, cake baking, reading, art and writing, or a loving nothingness. Knit a new-born hat, walk a beautiful park, eat whatever, whenever, and fall deep into the arms of lush vibrant wonderment. Sleep all you can.

There is fun too in this time. There is joy in taking walks and feeling twinges that may or may not be the surges of labour starting. There is pleasure in eating hot spicy curry, if you like curry (and I love curry so very much!), to attempt to kickstart labour. There is joy in hilarious great big and awkward hope-filled pregnancy sex. In many respects, your baby taking their time is an opportunity for working through tried and tested methods of bringing them out. In my experience, these are all hilarious and often abject failures. There can be a lightness to this stage, fused with expectation and emboldened with the most ridiculous hope that maybe this next slice of pineapple might solve the situation!

There is luck in your baby coming later than expected because you have not only that extra time, but the magical air of knowing it could happen any minute. For me this has meant moving into a portal of energy that is quite unique to any other moment in my life. It is a whimsical passageway of deep knowing, fused with absolute uncertainty, and whilst that may sound rather uneasy, in my experience it has always been rather scrumptious.

Renounce control and hand over to the timing that is, and always has been, something more perfect than your heart and mind can summon.

 ## Meditation: *The Meadow*

Play beautiful music and lie or sit in whatever way is most comfortable, ensuring your belly is supported. This meditation is designed to bring on deep rest and, if necessary, sleep. Breathing as deeply as comfortable, take a moment to connect to the inner world, to the babe in your womb, the ache of your joints, the flow of your body, the buzz of breath and blood and hope and expectation. Let it all just be, synchronising into the moment peacefully.

Bring yourself into the most beautiful meadow you can imagine, abundant with springy long grass, wildflowers, birds and pretty insects. This is a space to choose to be in, allowing everything else to drop away. Watch the clouds overhead and conjure the feeling of sun and breeze on your skin. There is nothing to do, nowhere to be, the simplicity of existence is all...

In this space take a moment to call on any inner wisdom to bubble up. Don't force it, or have expectations of what it may sound, feel or look like. If you are comfortable you may wish to contact the soul of your child directly, not with requests or demands, but simply to share some love, to remind them that you have their heart in your loving hands and are looking forward to meeting them. Fuse with their energy and remember that you as parent are holding space and safety for this tiny spirit.

Lay amongst the grasses and watch as the birds chase overhead, and even as the sun starts to set, leaving the sky open to a delight of pinpoint lights, shooting stars and indigo darkness.

Rest deeply and know that you are held. Be here as long as you wish.

 ## Soulful Practice: *Patience*

Patience is, and always has been, the most difficult spiritual practice. We want everything yesterday, and when we get it, we want the next thing: the next goal post or ticked box. Put all of that aside and move into the flow of what is. Impatience brings nothing but stress and frustration. This is the moment to place aware and loving boundaries between you and anybody else who may be impatient to meet your little one. Do not succumb to fearful talk or stories of others who have not been in your shoes. Listen to the guidance of the professionals supporting you, but always take time to reflect on the motives and personal narratives that underpin it.

Be fully with the clarity of love and the surrender to divine timing. Patience is a lesson that will visit you again and again in parenthood as in life. Learning to be with the moment now, as it is, really digging into this space, is a powerful mission and one that will support you and all you are becoming.

 ## Creative Practice: *Abundance*

This extended birth portal is a heightened time, and I encourage you to make the most of any senses that are flaring and flowing within you. Be abundantly with yourself and create as you see fit. Cake is great. Art is colourful and inspired. Writing is devotional and ecstatic. The garden is, if you can get to the ground, a pungent place to exert some energies. Books are calling to be read, and there is joy in some serious binging of your favourite shows. Movement is vital and necessary. You get to be right here, right now, in ways never previously experienced. Consider what you can do with this time, knowing it is limited, and with all of life brewing within.

Do what you wanna do. Simple. This is perhaps the last chance for a little while before you have your babe in arms and are busy with care and birth recovery. Do as you like, as you please, or not at all... Your creativity may look like binge-watching TV or trying a variety of hot curries to see if any of them prompt labour. It really doesn't matter. Be extra permissive with yourself right now. Be a creative sloth, be slovenly and lazy, make an art of that.

Some women experience a burst of energy at this time, if so, do whatever you desire with it. In my first pregnancy I used the last weeks to create cakes on a loop and paint slightly questionable pictures of nature. It was fun, and I filled my moments with light. So do, or do not do, at your pleasure!

If your body is tired and you are struggling with this time, then now can be a fruitful time to rest, to dream, to daydream and explore arising inner magic. The abundance does not miss you even if your body cannot express itself through art, dance, movement or words right now. Let the abundance of this moment be explored internally. Take long baths or showers, have conversations with friends that take you to new places and understandings. Creativity sparks even from bed rest and aching joints. Allow this moment to be a time unto yourself even if the fullest expression of that is currently beyond you.

 ## Journal Prompts

- How do I usually respond to the unexpected?

- Do I (or those who love me best) consider me patient?

- What do I usually fill space or time with? How might I choose differently now?

- Whose narratives do I need to detach from into order to fully enjoy this moment?

 Affirmation: *Every moment that passes has purpose. I relinquish any need to create or control this time.*

BIRTH

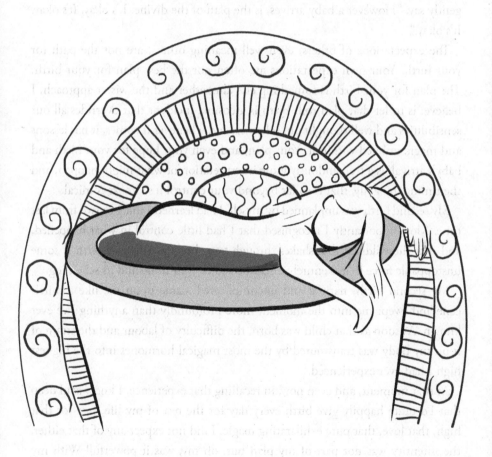

Birth is wild and tempestuous, and it bows to nobody. Even in the most spectacularly controlled medical circumstances, surprises can take place. Birth is perhaps your first real experience of the wild living itself out through your tamed body, blustery, unkempt and billowing with love. Birth in its true rawness defies description.

My first birth was induced, which was problematic for me as it was not what I planned. A fight began between my head and heart which distracted me from giving over to the moment. I fought long and hard for a 'natural' birth and when it didn't come, I devoured myself with guilt and shame. That baby's birth was perfect, despite it being massively off-plan, she is perfect.

As I look back on it now I want to hold my own sweet self and soothe her and gently say, "However a baby arrives, is the plan of the divine. It's okay. It's okay. It's okay."

The expectations of others, even well-meaning others, are not the path for your birth. Your own expectations are often not the best plan for your birth. The plan for your birth is something else altogether and the wisest approach, I believe, is to let that plan roll. Birth is a cosmic incident that overrides all our sensibilities and well thought out schemes, and whenever it comes, it has lessons and magic imbued within it. Your plan, and even your hope for your birth and baby's arrival, is a tremendously loose interpretation of what might happen, and the timing, by golly, that is so far beyond your control it's almost comical.

My second birth was unplanned by myself. I had learned a thing or two from last time. Most importantly I recognised that I had little control in what happened, and that the wildness that shakes through your body as you give birth is some unstoppable force that is entirely disconnected to your mind and its scheming.

My second birth, natural and uncomplicated, came upon me like a hurricane and swept me into the moment more profoundly than anything I've ever known. As soon as that child was born, the difficulty of labour and the strain of it on my body was transmuted by the most magical hormones into the highest high I had ever experienced.

At that moment, and even now, in recalling that experience, I know soul deep that I'd quite happily give birth every day for the rest of my life, just for that high, that love, that pure exhilarating magic. I did not expect any of that either, the intensity was not part of my plan but, oh my, was it powerful! With my second birth I didn't try to attain some perfect birth, there was no plan, no music list, no candles, it was me, my body, and the intensity and rawness of the moment was a triumph.

My third birth kept itself mysterious till the last minute. For a long time, natural birth looked problematic due to baby's breach position. When that naturally re-solved itself, I toyed with the plan for a home birth, but decided against it for sev-eral reasons that included personal intuition, but also the wise words of a midwife who spoke with great clarity to my head and heart and in relation to my personal circumstances. I attempted a little control and undertook some acupuncture with the hopes to nudge baby out naturally, alongside several failed cervical membrane sweeps. I declined induction at one point. Accepted it at another – booked in for a slightly later date. I hoped hard that a full blue moon might do the trick…

This third pregnancy had us in a place of limbo like never previously known, constantly making several sets of plans for every day to consider what may, or may not, happen. Birth being a huge unknown becomes exceptionally more tangled and uncertain as a process when you are low on childcare and with school age children (who had only that week gone back to school and the first year of high school after the summer break). The inability to focus on anything but what the moment offered was immense. I felt ill prepared, out of touch with the looming birth and surprisingly sweaty. Other matters took over: baby's position was off, my cervix wasn't primed, an intuitive voice within me at the age of forty-four years old and utterly exhausted started to drop words my way I had not considered.

It was at this point that all my expectations of the situation and myself dropped. I started to entertain a planned caesarean section. This came up within me naturally and was not an option being presented or pushed. Immediately the weight and pressure lifted, and I felt a return to a more soulful self, a calmer self, a self who relented and released what she thought 'should' happen and began to explore something I never believed I would. As a 'soulful' writer of spiritual books, it seemed I ought really to be having a 'certain kind of birth'. When I entered the realms of something other than that, the fight was not with anything other than myself, and the expectations I had. Yet I had been surrounded by cae-sarean positive women my whole pregnancy, those who had found their births beautiful, spiritual and celebratory.

I took time to drop into what felt right, what felt soulful. It wasn't what I thought it would be. It wasn't the home birth or wrestling with my timeline to conjure a natural birth (though I would welcome that should it befall me), it was not the very limited induction I was being offered that may or may not prove effective and required me being prepped for theatre no matter what. I sliced through all the things I thought I wanted and decided to take a path I'd never contemplated. I booked in a caesarean section based on the clarity of my heart, and in doing so recognised that so often in life the biggest problem is the fight within.

Despite this decision being so very surprising, I found myself on the eve of that elective section writing this, and healing a wound put in place from my first birth. That wound was one of trying to fit in to one stream of thought, the fight to produce my child a specific way, and feeling lost between the mêlée of two systems (natural and medical). Neither of those sets of options feeling entirely safe, neither of them knowing me, like I now know me.

I released all words shared with me about birth from all sides of the beautiful act. I sat in peace with a decision I hadn't planned to make and found my soulfulness not in any one way, not in a performance, not in efforts or actions, but in sourcing and knowing what felt best, for me, at a pivotal moment. This is my soulful pregnancy made manifest in one final life-giving choice: the ability to look inward and to know that for whatever reason, one option shines brighter, bolder and more comfortable than any other. I am gifting myself a choice I was not able to make or even see some eleven years ago. I am experiencing my own clarity and permitting it.

This shiny and unexpected choice resulted in a beautiful boy whose presence feels like magic, light and purpose. His coming to this planet was an adventure, his being here is the real gift.

A healthy child brought earthside is a miracle and the divine provides so many ways for that to happen in our modern world. You can't get it wrong; it is beyond you. You are a conduit not the mega mind. Birth is not in your power or choice to mess up. It never was. So let your plans fall to the side and trust that whatever comes, be that natural birth, caesarean section, or a one-hour labour with a babe born in the back of an Uber, all is as it should be. Open your heart and mind to the divine power afoot and the flow of something that has nothing to do with what you (or anyone) thinks should happen.

Whilst it is important to relent and release when it comes to birth, there is equally so much power in being deeply prepared and ready to stand your ground. You can allow events to flow, whilst also being an active participant in decisions being made and the requirements you may have. Have your birth plan handy and ensure that anyone attending the birth as your partner is aware of its details. Whilst some of this may get lost to what happens, there will be many empowering elements that can be non-negotiable or worked with flexibly. Building a team around your birth in preparation, to speak with or for you, is vital, so trust that, whilst birth has its own plan, you can steer the course somewhat, and your birthing partner, midwife or doula can advocate for you at your request.

Liberate yourself to birth in exactly the way you birth when it happens. This, for me, is empowerment. It is empowering to get on the ride and let it take you, with trust, with love and with a readiness to take what comes and/or change your heart and mind as the situation flows. Let the moments of birth become you and pray, not for some perfected and manicured version of your baby coming into being, but for their health, for yours, and for the magnitude of the portal you walk through towards the rest of your life. This is birth, a labyrinth of nature, of challenge, of growth and desire, culminating, you pray, in meeting the next love of your life. That is all. That is everything. I wish you all the power and clarity…

 # Meditation: *Birth*

It is likely your birth may not allow for great long and luscious meditative ramblings. So, this is simple and can be engaged with no matter the type or style of birthing – you may wish to familiarise yourself with it in the time leading to birth (and use it alongside any other favourites from this book). Hopefully your many meditative practices over the last forty weeks have prepared you to be able to drop inwards and operate from a less 'surface' space.

Bring yourself to your breath, close your eyes, and go straight into your inner world, your inner experience. Go beyond the outward levels of contractions, surges, pain, surrounding events and discomfort, seek inwardly to find a still point, a place unaffected by the birthing that is occurring.

Breathe deeply into this place. As you recognise the essential and everlasting point of 'control' inwardly, imagine this place expanding. Allow this small pearl of stillness and peace to grow and bring with it soothing and calming properties.

Breathe into the peace within, giving it permission to comfort and hang beautifully within the moment, becoming a framework of stillness for you to hang all else upon. Recognise that you can have two experiences at once, the surface experience and whatever physicality and emotionality that this entails, but that you also welcome the inner peace, the internal loving observer, and ask this part of you to engage, to grow, to take up more space.

It may help to envision the internal peaceful space as a certain colour or even an object. You may locate it on your body, and find your attention pulled to that area, your hands, or the hands of helpers gently massaging this still point if that feels good. Breathe into this place with oils, incense and hope. You need not leave the room mentally as with some meditations, but rather, you can lean into all that is happening, whilst allowing for peaceful knowing to grow bigger and help carry you.

If you drop out of engagement with this still inward point, that is okay. You can remember to return whenever it feels easy and accessible. You may find that using words internally and externally helps, thinking or saying to yourself: "I go inwards to safety and stillness" or "I call on my inner stillness and strength."

Even just dropping this down to a fragment, a small key of connection may help, as you mutter and repeat to yourself: "stillness", "strength", even calling in divine assistance if it feels powerful.

Bring yourself back to this source of inner spiritual strength using breath and conscious will repeatedly. Whenever you feel connected let the connection expand, and as it drops away trust that this too is necessary. Let the waves of connection grow stronger, as at the same time baby comes closer to Earth and your arms.

 ## Soulful Practice:
Your Spiritual Birth Support

As you move towards birth it can be empowering to pinpoint a spiritual deity, a god or goddess, or some other fitting divine entity (angels, guides, power animals, flower totem) to be at your side as you birth. This may come from your spiritual experiences, religious background, or be a divine character you have engaged with and found helpful in the past or have discovered in this book. You may wish to research them and if they have any connection with life-bringing, parenthood, transformation and strength-giving. Whichever spiritual embodiment you feel called to will have so much to offer you, so trust the call.

As I step closer to my birth, I speak every night, before I fall asleep, to a whole team of spiritual helpers, asking them to step forward and be with me in this time. I call in guides, departed loved ones and ancestors, asking them to lend strength, courage and magic to however the next days and weeks play out. Just last night an image of one of my grandfathers came to mind as I was falling asleep, he was a great friend to children, and I took his appearance as evidence of his being around. Ask and see who finds a way to step forward...

Alongside this I spend time recalling the elements and making space for them in my heart, remembering how they support my existence, and have supported a billion birthing women throughout time before me.

You may wish to wear a piece of jewellery in their honour, or have a small statue, crystal, pebble or image dedicated to them tucked away with your hospital bag or birthing things. Give them permission before birth to infuse you with their highest and most helpful energies, and revisit this as needed during your birthing.

When in birth or anytime in the lead up to birth, you may wish to formally invite your soul team in using the following words...

"I invite my spiritual guides/angels/beloved ancestors/xxxx to attend this birth, to offer their power, support and skills to assist myself and baby."

Creative Practice: *Birth Creatively*

Birth may leave many of your creative practices in the dust, yet it is wise to keep an open mind concerning how your general creativity may be helpful. Creativity can arise in all life circumstances, and so something as simple as positioning, choice of entertainment during early labour or the way you interact with those in attendance can contain elements of the creative. Keep your mind and heart open to the opportunity to be creative, and to redefine the parameters of your birth accordingly. Here are a few examples...

- Think about your body position. Give yourself permission to move and take up stances that feel right for you during the different stages of labour: circle your hips, rock, sway, kneel, stand...

- Spend time, perhaps in early labour, or when moments grab you, thinking or talking to a partner about what the 'next day' might look and feel like. This will help shift the intensity, allowing you to recall that there is life waiting beyond this act. Indeed that this moment is essential for you to create the perceived future.

- Invoke creativity to keep yourself calm. You may wish to have handy a colouring book and pencils for use in a long slow labour. It may sound minor, but the soothing effect of gentle colouring is easily forgotten yet surprisingly powerful.

- Bless your body with good flavours and hydration. Call on helpers to provide the grapes, juice or chocolate – anything that feels essential to energy, as and when required.

- Sound. You may want to listen to music, chant, sing, shout or groan during birth. Let your sounds free.

- Endorphins and oxytocin (the love and pleasure hormones) are helpful in birthing, and some recommend kissing and gentle affection and touching with your partner. There are other ways to engage and elevate happy hormones, this might be music you love, food, having a favourite film on, or watching a hilarious comedian. There is no right or wrong here, and whilst making out with your partner might be one way, there are also so many other ways to raise a smile and equally help you feel earthed and grounded and in touch with hormones that might creatively elevate your experience.

Every turn of your birthing journey can engage your creative approach should you wish, so keep creativity in your arsenal of potential responses, decisions and actions as you bring your baby to Earth.

 ## Journal Prompts

- What am I good at in life and how might this skill be applied to birth?
- At this portal of change, what three feelings am I most engaging with? Are these helpful? If not, how might I shift them?
- What do I need right now and how can that need be served?
- Do I need to ask for help, reassurance, a cuddle? If yes, do so…

 Affirmation: *I welcome all that occurs to bring my child to me in health and love.*

FOURTH TRIMESTER

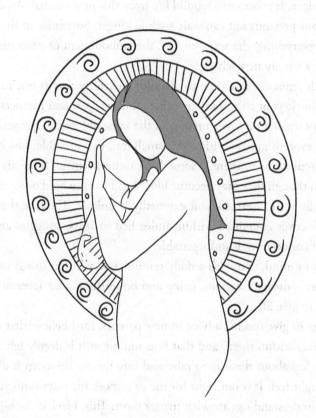

AND BEYOND

The fourth trimester is so-called because whilst your baby is no longer in the womb, they are still so fully dependent upon you and other caregivers. There is nothing like it: going from autonomy of mind and body, to becoming the essential life-support of another. For most people this is a shock to the system, and alongside hormones, post-natal depression and post-birth healing, the surprise of being so massively responsible can be deeply difficult. For me there is one answer which is both spiritual and ultimately rather sensible: surrender.

Surrender to what this is. Right now, there is no scraping back the remnants of what was before. It is better to rebuild life from this new normal. An attempt to return to your previous self can wait a while longer. Surrender to the intensity, the shift of everything, the way you feel, the embodiment of parenting and the demands of a wholly new schedule.

The fourth trimester is a time to abandon anything that is not in your immediate vicinity: your baby and any other children, pets and partners. Your life may feel very small for a time, a repeat of the same old feeds, changes, naps and interrupted everything. Yet within this smallness, this invisible, unseen time of newborn circumstances, there is something quite massive. These are days you won't forget, though they may become blurry and hard to hold onto; the feeling, the unworldly shift internally and externally is unique. The love that you will hopefully discover contained within, unleashed in tears, snuggles and blissful moments of connection, is unforgettable.

With this in mind, and with a daily reminder to self that this is not forever, the moments – dreary, hilarious, tiring and bountiful – are a fever of what it is to live, and to give life.

I don't like to give specific advice to new parents, for I believe that the expert they need lives within them, and that is as unique as it is deeply felt and intuitive. How I feel about the way to raise and care for my newborn is different to how you might feel. It is not right for me to impose my ways onto yours. Your developing understandings are what matter most. This, I feel, is the biggest challenge of early parenthood: the search inward to figure out what feels right. Then to give yourself permission to follow your inner guide.

This is your biggest mission. To figure out who you are as a parent, to steer clear of advice that doesn't work, and to become happy with your choices. It sounds simple, doesn't it? Yet we are subsumed in a culture that has strong opinions about everything from how you hold your baby, to how it is fed, to how you deal with their sleep and every other choice for the next eighteen years. Building strong foundations in favour of what works for you and your unique child is the structure that you may be seeking out within these first few months. Doubtless you will be encouraged in many directions by family, midwives, friends and your internet searches. My advice to every suggestion is for you to carefully consider: does it feel good, does it feel natural, does it feel loving, does it feel like mine?

The fourth trimester is a test of all that you are. It asks you to change so much within the daily dynamic of your life, and to go deep into the guts of self and figure out who you are becoming and how you will choose to run the show. Go easy. You may not get it all right quickly. It is a passage to be gently fathomed. Mistakes will lead to better answers, and fear will eventually give way to inner knowing if you allow it. This is a time to forge yourself through milky nights and gut-wrenching emotion. It is a time to rest and cease action, whilst simultaneously being on guard, responsive and attentive.

The fourth trimester is a rebirth of you as you begin the path to leading another into what it is to live, to love and to exist within connection. May you have the courage to find your way and follow it boldly. May you have the perspective to recognise that what you have known in your life so far need not follow through to this next journey, that from here you get to redesign the patterns in your life and your familial line. May you wind your way through your days knowing you were made for this moment, and you bring to it every wisdom, and all the potential your child (and your inner child) needs.

The First Few Days Post-Partum

People suggest that life stops when you have a small baby in your arms, and perhaps you pick it up again later. I do not fully agree. The intensity of early days parenting is not a stop sign. It may be a 'find a new route' sign but does not need to be closure. I have found that this time is fertile rather than stagnant, and even if I am just making notes for the future, or experiencing some gorgeous soulful connection, my creativity and spirituality remain very close.

I found moments of great spirituality in feeding my children. I could have been

distracted from this by binge watching or scrolling my
phone over baby's head (which I did too, of course
I did). Yet being in darkness, soothing or feeding or
singing lullabies to a very small child, is deeply sacred.
What arises here may surprise you. I recall resting with my
babes in our first few weeks, losing myself to the cocoon of all
that is brought to our arms: the tiredness, the love, the magic,
the innocence, the smell of their soft heads. Sitting on your sofa
for hour upon end with a child in your arms is a meditation. As you lose yourself
to their feel, their softness and smell, things rise from within: ideas, thoughts,
love, insights. This time, so visibly short, can be as expansive as your soul, if you
allow it.

Meditation: *Resting in a Cocoon*

The space of the fourth trimester is one of intensity. There is the intensity of
love, and the perhaps unexpected powerful hold your babe has upon you. There
is nothing like it in the world. In whatever way this intensity shows up for you,
it is important that you create safe spaces within it to give over to the burgeoning
connection between you and your baby, but to also take a moment to yourself.

This meditation expects little from you, because I am aware that time is too
engaged and busy to be put aside. Indeed, it is probably best undertaken with
child in arms, perhaps feeding or sleeping, and allows for you to recentre and
calibrate your energies.

To undertake this meditation all you need is your breath and a few minutes.
Gently close your eyes, whilst sitting (be cautious not to fall asleep if the baby is
in your arms) and breathe deeply. Imagine briefly that you and your child are in
a cocoon. Rock gently back and forth, perhaps humming or singing a favoured
lullaby. Let this be your all. You are the cocoon for baby, just as this moment,
the breath, the peacefulness is a cocoon for you. Be lost to the moment. Allow
yourself to be exactly as you are and to feel what is necessary. Let emotions surface, or simply be in total cocooned presence.

When you are ready, bring your attention back to the wider space around you,
open your eyes and continue to rest, feed or be with your newborn.

Soulful Practice: *Savouring the Moment*

This week's Soulful Practice is the easiest. Gaze at your baby, whisper in their ear, take deep long breaths of their unique smell. Speak to them gently, or sing them a song, marvel and wonder at their fingers and toes. There is no requirement to do or be anything other than the situation that is. Heighten the moment and really live within it, this time passes quickly.

Creative Practice: *Capturing the Moment*

In the weeks following my births I try to do the following to capture precious memories.

Write down your birth story. If you feel ready and able, the details of your birth story can be captured whilst fresh in your mind. This will help you to make sense and memories of them, and is also a beautiful thing for you to share with your child at some time in the future. It may be that you write a list of notes or salient memories. If the birth was difficult, you may focus on the lead up to birth and the feeling the first time they were placed in your arms, or when you took them home. You can recall the reactions of other people when they first met the baby, alongside a list of any gifts they received, or kind loving words that were spoken in their honour.

Take photographs of your baby with people who love them. These are to be treasured in the future and help your child feel connected, welcomed, and wanted. I have enjoyed keeping a private record of my children's adventures from babyhood onward using Instagram. My kids love perusing this, in the same way I used to love looking at family photo albums as a child.

Start a little journal for them. With my first daughter I indulged a full diary of her every action and my loving feelings for her. Admittedly by the time my second was born, there was less time and energy to write things down, but I tried and made notes for her to look at one day.

Now is the perfect time **to take prints of their tiny hands and feet** to remember how small they once were. Use non-toxic poster paint to take prints and use them to decorate thank you cards as well as for a keepsake for your baby album or to display framed on the wall.

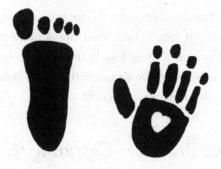

Journal Prompts

- What do I most want to remember from this precious time?

- What has surprised me the most?

- What support do I need and how can I ask for it?

- How has life changed, and how am I handling this?

 Affirmation: *I give myself fully to these precious moments.*

Motherhood as Creative Portal

Pregnancy is not alone in being a time when our soulful and creative inklings surge. I have found that being a parent allows for fits and spurts of creativity and spirituality in amongst the mundane and domesticity of everyday life. This doesn't mean you should birth your baby and immediately take to an easel. Rather, it's important to recognise that your connection to inner creativity and spiritual longing should not stop because you have given birth.

The early years of your child's life whilst so intensive, are also a breeding ground for fertile ideas and insight. It may not always be the time to put those thoughts into full action, however, it is a space of great potential. Much of that potential is seized when we choose to make room for it.

Making room can be as simple as giving yourself fully to the moment, herein, in this immediate now space, there can be a great deal that arises. As our bodies heal, and baby grows, we may find time to grasp small windows to consider this even further.

Do not presume that this part of your life will look like anything you have experienced before, or that it might lack your usual veracity. Keep a notepad handy, some pens and an open mind. When the moment takes you, and a thought, vision or idea arises, write it down. Doodle yourself alive whilst baby rests.

It is in the aftermath of my children's births that I have found unexpected spaces to create. This work doesn't look like a nine-to-five, it comes in very short segments of time. I am writing this as my seven-year-old has a telephone call with her grandma. This may give me five minutes, or maybe half an hour, but I was in the mood, so I grabbed the laptop and let words come. If it had been yesterday, I would have probably lain in bed and done nothing. I give myself permission to be with creativity when I feel like it. This means it's never forced, I'm not compelled to hours of writing, and so I can take blips in time and fill them how I wish.

When your child is old enough, have them join you. I've done art with my kids since they were old enough to get stuck in. I created a deck of seventy-eight tarot cards (my *Cosmic Mother Tarot*) with my four-year-old in the moments that my newborn slept. It kept us entertained, gave us a focus and helped us to bond. I've done the potato printing, the hand drawing, the scribbles, and paint chucking and paper folding alongside them (it has taught me a great deal). Sometimes, whilst they make a mess with watercolours or pencil work, I try my hand at a portrait of the dog, or a vase of flowers. In togetherness we rise, and the lesson I hope they receive is that art, creativity and expression is for life, and we must always find a way.

Find your way. Keep your tools close. Maybe you will use them, perhaps you won't. I promise, however, that this stepping into your children's world is also them stepping into yours. Together you can envision and embody a life of sacred, creative expression.

 # Meditation: *Being You*

In the early years of motherhood it is easy to lose track of who we are beyond our mothering role. It is often good to take a moment to remember that this is one season of our lives.

Slip into your comfortable space, take a breath, and open your heart. Literally envision your heart opening as if it has a door or windows, release any dusty old energy, and spill wide to open to the new.

You might like to imagine a bright light making its way from the cosmos directly into your heart, carrying with it the energy of your essential being. This is the version of you that is celestial, ever true and full of itself in the best possible way. It is full fruited and undiluted. Let this energy flow into your heart, from here, imagine the heartbeat carrying this pure version of self all around your body, your cells and your spirit.

Welcome this energy in. Feel yourself in technicolour, uninterrupted and full. Imagine that the cracks and fractures of your current life are healed and made whole. You are yourself in totality. Anything that does not belong to you is pushed out, forced away. You are becoming yourself as your energy floods and returns.

Take a moment to speak with yourself. Who are you now? Who do you wish to be? How will you choose to grow moving forward?

Welcome yourself home.

When you feel complete and returned, take a deep breath and be with your own power as you return to everyday life.

Soulful Practice:
Start a Spiritual Diary

I have found that as I had my children, roads opened to intriguing spiritual understandings, visions, dreams and coincidences. I wish I had written these down, particularly as some of these related directly to my kids, including intriguing and magical things that they said and did.

A spiritual journal is a good place to record your hopes, desires and the intensity of situations and emotions. It is a sacred space that allows for all your parts to be seen. Source a lovely journal and good pen, add these into your 'creative kit' (see below). Let the portal of birth become the passage to actively interacting with your spiritual happenings as and when they arrive.

Creative Practice: *Creative Kit*

Create a handy kit bag of spiritual and creative tools for these early months, so that you can access it easily, create where you are and stash it away quickly afterwards. It doesn't need to be anything too complex, think pens, paper, your spiritual journal, a colouring book, your handy knitting needles or crochet hook, your Kindle or a couple of books, crystals, essential oils, tarot cards, incense and a lighter or whatever else feels doable. Keep this bag alongside your baby's things, or next to your favourite spot on the sofa, dig it out on occasion when time is on your side and reconnect to the creative and soulful aspects of yourself.

Don't forget about your phone. You will doubtless have it around you through those early days. Recognise how this can be a distraction…or useful creative tool. Use it to create a photographic diary or capture interesting moments that sit outside of the usual images we see of babies. Now might be a good time to set up a new photographic account, get hold of some intriguing photo apps or open a folder in your phone ready to fill with creative shots of your early life with baby.

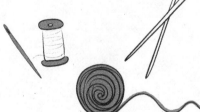

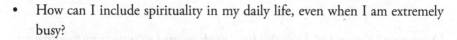

Journal Prompts

- How can I include spirituality in my daily life, even when I am extremely busy?
- How might I engage my creativity frequently (consider ways of life, choices, relationships and personal expression).
- My prayer, at this moment is…
- My creativity feeds me in the following ways…
- My spirituality fuels me in this manner…

 Affirmation: *I welcome new ways to engage and understand all parts of myself.*

Closing

In closing this book, it is vital that you recognise your journey has only just begun. So much weight is placed upon pregnancy as a magical state of creation. And it is, but it might be more accurate to say that the real time of creativity starts when your baby is in your arms.

My words to you as you embark upon this journey are, yes, you will make errors, and do things you regret. That is the state of being human. The magic lies in your ability to continue to grow, alongside your child. Just as you tutor your child in life, so you can allow them to school you. As with every error, there is always a recourse, a way of being better, a lived apology and an ever-extending of love that showers you and them in protection and possibility. Begin this journey with a fluidity and flexibility that allows for you to lead and to be led, to love and to accept love, to see and honour their needs, just as you learn to see and honour your own.

The dance that is born when your child is birthed is one of dependence, devotion and the opportunity to become so much more. It's not easy. Often, it's not that hard either. Sometimes it is delicious, divine and all that you will ever really need. It's a flow and a constant realignment: the tempo changes the moment you rest easy and believe that things have hit a rhythm you can move to, the tune will shift and throw a faster dance beat at you. You adapt – you must – and the new grooves can feel just as good once your hips find their way. For this reason alone, parenthood requires all of you, all at once, especially in these early days. Keep track of the beat, and yes, of course, at times, you get to change the tune and introduce new moves to the dancefloor.

Please do revisit this book over the years. Every week of the pregnancy journey contains areas of growth that stay relevant throughout life. It may be that opening on a random page, in times of need, will bring you just the right practice or meditation, or words of comfort, as you navigate the path to adulthood with your child.

As I have stated previously, the only real advice I or anyone should ever give you, is do what feels good, do what feels right to you, do what feels like love and disregard anything that does not fit those criteria. This is your time to step up, to become the elder, to put all your lived experiences and inner knowing to the test. If that inner knowing feels in short supply, trust that this parenting journey will bring it in buckets, and that you are capable of receiving and transmuting it into your family with love, ease and care.

I wish you a soulful life of happiness, courage, self-compassion, inner knowing and all the love this parenting path can possibly offer.

Alice

Acknowledgments

Bowie – beautiful boy. I cannot wait to meet you and grow with your wonderful spirit and energy. This book is a testament to you (and your sisters) but it wouldn't have happened without you – thank you for joining us.

My daughters, Ivy and Clover, for teasing me mercilessly throughout this pregnancy, being true little soul friends to me and each other, with a good fat dollop of rebellion, noise, insanity and spirit. Never ever change, you are the light.

Mabbles, thank you for being a reflection, and loving me, believing in me, and encouraging my creativity regardless. Love you all!

Much thanks to Lucy Pearce for having me and this book on Womancraft. *Soulful Pregnancy* feels extra magical thanks to your steering, belief and wise editing. And thanks to those behind the scenes at Womancraft who help pull this all together.

Love to my Rebel Heart Coven, Niki and Kizzy, a true meeting of souls that has been all the Three of Cups vibes and without which my life and work would not be so spirited and abundant.

Special thanks to Niki Cotton for the incredible cover art and willingness to sit with and interpret my (confusing) requests.

To my family and friends. Love and thanks for all your never-ending support and inspiration.

About the Author

Alice's work is renowned for providing an earthy and everyday perspective on a spiritual life, making the divine accessible, welcoming and fun to anyone seeking it.

Author of five published books on spirituality and tarot and creator of two card decks including *Rebel Heart*. In 2023 she was voted *Kindred Spirit* magazine's MBS Author of the Year. Alice's work and articles have been shared worldwide and have appeared in print, online, radio and television.

Alongside her written work and card deck creation, Alice teaches and shares spirituality with a modern female audience through her Cosmic Sisterhood, newsletter and frequent workshops which she both hosts and attends at the request of other workshop hosts to share the unique power of tarot and oracle cards.

Based in Middle England she is devoted to a life of creativity, spiritual exploration, family and everyday magic.

alicegrist.com   Facebook/alicegristtarot

Instagram/alicegrist   TikTok/alicegrist_tarot

Other Books and Card Decks by the Author

Rebel Heart Tarot (Card Deck) – Welbeck, 2022

The Book of Tarot – Piatkus, 2020

Dirty & Divine: a transformative journey through tarot – Womancraft Publishing, 2017

Cosmic Mother Tarot – self-published, 2017

Dear Poppyseed: A Soulful Momma's Pregnancy Journal – John Hunt Publishing, 2013

The High Heeled Guide to Spiritual Living – John Hunt Publishing, 2011

The High Heeled Guide to Enlightenment – John Hunt Publishing, 2009

About the Cover Artist

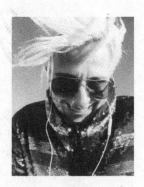

Niki is a contemporary Welsh visual artist working from a studio & gallery space on the coast of North Wales. Her practice stretches across many mediums including collage, painting, printmaking, sculpture, performance, textiles and photography.

As a Generation X'er, Niki finds herself referencing the pop culture and music of the 80's and 90's where she grew up, whilst absorbing the rebellious nature of Punk and the brashness of Americana. Having just completed an MA in Fine Art, Niki is occupied with thoughts of what it is to be a woman in the 21st Century and with the advent of children and motherhood – the fracturing and fragmenting of self that occurs and the endlessness of domestic drudgery.

A visual voice that echoes the madness of juggling an over-full life where she says she feels like a cake that doesn't have quite enough slices to go around all the people at the party.

About Womancraft

Womancraft Publishing was founded on the revolutionary vision that women and words can change the world. We act as midwife to transformational women's words that have the power to challenge, inspire, heal and speak to the silenced aspects of ourselves, empowering our readers to actively co-create cultures that value and support the female and feminine. Our books have been #1 Amazon bestsellers in many categories, as well as Nautilus and Women's Spirituality Award winners.

As we find ourselves in a time where old stories, old answers and ways of being are losing their authority and relevance, we at Womancraft are actively looking for new ways forward. Our books ask important questions. We aim to share a diverse range of voices, of different ages, backgrounds, sexual orientations and neurotypes, seeking every greater diversity, whilst acknowledging our limitations as a small press.

Whilst far from perfect, we are proud that in our small way, Womancraft is walking its talk, living the new paradigm in the crumbling heart of the old: through financially empowering creative people, through words that honour the Feminine, through healthy working practices, and through integrating business with our lives, and rooting our economic decisions in what supports and sustains our natural environment. We are learning and improving all the time. I hope that one day soon, what we do is seen as nothing remarkable, just the norm.

We work on a full circle model of giving and receiving: reaching backwards, supporting Treesisters' reforestation projects and the UNHCR girls' education fund, and forwards via Worldreader, providing e-books at no-cost to education projects for girls and women in developing countries. We donate many paperback copies to education projects and women's libraries around the world. We speak from our place within the circle of women, sharing our vision, and encouraging them to share it onwards, in ever-widening circles.

We are honoured that the Womancraft community is growing internationally year on year, seeding red tents, book groups, women's circles, ceremonies and classes into the fabric of our world. Join the revolution! Sign up to the mailing list at womancraftpublishing.com and find us on social media for exclusive offers:

 womancraftpublishing   womancraft_publishing

Signed copies of all titles available from womancraftpublishing.com

Dirty & Divine

Alice Grist

A tarot-led vision quest to reclaiming your femininity in all its lucid and colourful depths.

There is something sacred within you, in all that you are and all that you do. In a mix of you that is everyday dirty, and spiritually divine, there is something so perfect, something more. Welcome to your journey back home; to your dirty, divine passage back to you.

Wherever you are, whether beginner or seasoned tarot practitioner, *Dirty & Divine* is written for you, to accompany you on a powerful personal intuitive journey to plumb the depths of your existence and encompass the spectrum of wisdom that the cards can offer.

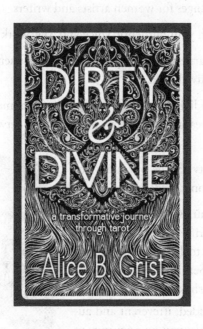

Creatrix

Lucy H. Pearce

Creatrix is more than just a fancy name for a female artist. She is artist plus... artist plus priestess, artist plus healer, artist plus activist: her work has both sacred and worldly dimensions. She is an energy worker first and foremost, weaving energy into form, colour, words and sound, in order to transform herself and those her creations touch.

What does it mean to live a life in service to your creativity, and in direct connection to the creative source?

In this, her ninth book, Lucy H. Pearce, award-winning author of *Burning Woman, Medicine Woman* and *The Rainbow Way* shares...

- Powerful practical insight into all parts of The Creative Way.

- The unique challenges for women artists and writers.

- How to align with your authentic voice and The Work that calls you.

- Techniques for harnessing your powerful creative energy and dealing with fear, anxiety, creative blocks.

- How to earn your living creatively: building a social media platform, working sustainably, creating multiple income streams, networking when socially anxious...

- How our creativity can be our most potent transformational medicine.

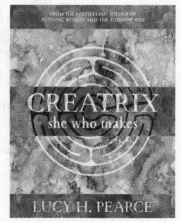

With Creative Inquiries and Practices, this interactive book is written for all those that must create in order to live: for the Highly Creative, the Highly Sensitive, the multi-passionate, for those that shake when they share...

Soulful, serious-minded, irreverent and authentic, let Creatrix take you on a journey to the heart of your creative soul.